CLINICAL AND EXPERIMENTAL STUDIES IN IMMUNOTHERAPY

CLINICAL AND EXPERIMENTAL STUDIES IN IMMUNOTHERAPY

Proceedings of an international symposium held at

The 13th International Congress of Chemotherapy

Vienna, September, 1983

Editors:

Takashi Hoshino
Fukui Medical School
Fukui, Japan

Atsushi Uchida
Paterson Laboratories
Christie Hospital and
Holt Radium Institute
Manchester, U.K.

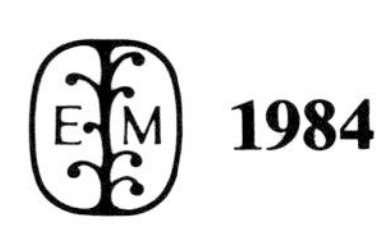

1984

Excerpta Medica, Amsterdam-Princeton-Geneva-Tokyo

Current Clinical Practice Series No.17
ISBN Excerpta Medica 4-900392-25-1

Publisher: Excerpta Medica

Offices: P.O. Box 1126
1000-BC Amsterdam

28, Chemin Colladon
Geneva

P.O. Box 3085
Princeton, N.J. 08540

15-23 Nishi Azabu, 4-Chome
Minato-ku, Tokyo

Printed in Japan

List of contributors

Tibor BAKACS
National Institute of Oncology
Budapest XII
Rath Gyorgy u. 7–9
Hungary

Jean P. BUREAU
Laboratoire d'Histologie
et Immunogénétique
Faculté de Médecine
Nimes-Montpellier
30 000 Nimes
France

Michael A. CHIRIGOS
Immunopharmacology Section
Biological Therapeutics Branch
Biological Response Modifiers Program
Div. of Cancer Treatment
National Cancer Institute
Frederick Cancer Research Facility
P.O.Box B, Frederick, Maryland 21701
U.S.A.

Francesco COLOTTA
Istituto di Ricerche Farmacologiche
Mario Negri
Via Eritrea, 62, 20157 Milano
Italy

Didier CUPISSOL
Service de Chimio-Immunothérapie
et Laboratoire d'Immunopharmacologie
des Tumeurs
INSERM U-236, ERA-CNRS no 844
Centre Paul Lamarque
BP 5054, 34 033
Montpellier-Cédex
France

Vukašin DANGUBIĆ
Institute for Lung Diseases
Military Medical Academy
Grnotravska bb
11002 Belgrade
Yugoslavia

Aleksandar DIJIĆ
Institute for Experimental Medicine
Military Medical Academy
Grnotravska bb
11002 Belgrade
Yugoslavia

Takashi FUJIMURA	The First Dept. of Surgery Kyushu University School of Medicine 3–1–1 Maidashi, Higashi-ku, Fukuoka 812 Japan
Takashi HOSHINO	Dept. of Immunology and Parasitology Fukui Medical School Shimoaizuki, Matsuoka-cho, Yoshida-gun Fukui 910–11 Japan
Osamu ICHIMURA	Research Laboratories I Chugai Pharmaceutical Co., Ltd. 3–41–8 Takada, Toshima-ku, Tokyo 171 Japan
Takashi IWA	Dept. of Surgery Kanazawa University School of Medicine 13–1 Takara-machi, Kanazawa 920 Japan
Mitsuo KATANO	Dept. of Surgery Saga Medical School Nabeshima-cho, Saga 840–01 Japan
Masato KATO	The First Dept. of Surgery Kyushu University School of Medicine 3–1–1 Maidashi, Higashi-ku, Fukuoka 812 Japan
Masatoshi KATO	The First Dept. of Surgery Kyushu University School of Medicine 3–1–1 Maidashi, Higashi-ku, Fukuoka 812 Japan
Jin-Pok KIM	Dept. of Surgery College of Medicine Seoul National University Hospital 28 Yunkun-Dong, Chongro-ku Seoul 110 Korea
Sang-Joon KIM	Dept. of Surgery College of Medicine Seoul National University Hospital 28 Yunkun-Dong, Chongro-ku Seoul 110 Korea

Yoon Berm KIM	Dept. of Microbiology and Immunology University of Health Sciences The Chicago Medical School 3333 Green Bay Road North Chicago, Illinois 60064 U.S.A.
Ian KIMBER	Immunology Section ICI, Central Toxicology Laboratory Alderley Park, Macclesfield Cheshire, SK10 4TJ U.K.
Nada KOLAŠINOVIĆ	Institute for Experimental Medicine Military Medical Academy Grnotravska bb 11002 Belgrade Yugoslavia
Kohki KONOMI	The First Dept. of Surgery Kyushu University School of Medicine 3-1-1 Maidashi, Higashi-ku, Fukuoka 812 Japan
Desa LILIĆ	Institute for Experimental Medicine Military Medical Academy Grnotravska bb 11002 Belgrade Yugoslavia
Alberto MANTOVANI	Istituto di Ricerche Farmacologiche Mario Negri Via Eritrea, 62, 20157 Milano Italy
Michael MICKSCHE	Institute for Applied and Experimental Oncology University of Wien A1010 Wien Austria
Tadanori MIYATA	The First Dept. of Surgery Kyushu University School of Medicine 3-1-1 Maidashi, Higashi-ku, Fukuoka 812 Japan
Michael MOORE	Div. of Immunology, Paterson Laboratories Christie Hospital and Holt Radium Institute Manchester M20 9BX U.K.

Toshiaki OSAWA
Div. of Chemical Toxicology and Immunochemistry
Faculty of Pharmaceutical Sciences
University of Tokyo
7-3-1 Hongo, Bunkyo-ku, Tokyo 113
Japan

Jae-Gahb PARK
Dept. of Surgery
College of Medicine
Seoul National University Hospital
28 Yunkun-Dong, Chongro-ku
Seoul 110
Korea

Tohru SAITO
Immunopharmacology Section
Biological Therapeutics Branch
Biological Response Modifiers Program
Div. of Cancer Treatment
National Cancer Institute
Frederick Cancer Research Facility
P.O.Box B, Frederick, Maryland 21701
U.S.A

Masaki SAKATA
The First Dept. of Surgery
Kyushu University School of Medicine
3-1-1 Maidashi, Higashi-ku, Fukuoka 812
Japan

Bernard SERROU
Service de Chimio-Immunothérapie
et Laboratoire d'Immunopharmacologie des Tumeurs
INSERM U-236, ERA-CNRS no 844
Centre Paul Lamarque
BP 5054, 34 033
Montpellier-Cédex
France

Enzo SORESI
Niguarda Hospital
Piazza Ospedale Maggiore
Milan
Italy

Yutaka SUGAWARA
Research Laboratories I
Chugai Pharmaceutical Co., Ltd.
3-41-8 Takada, Toshima-ku, Tokyo 171
Japan

Seikichi SUZUKI
Research Laboratories I
Chugai Pharmaceutical Co., Ltd.
3-41-8 Takada, Toshima-ku, Tokyo 171
Japan

James E. TALMADGE — Preclinical Screening Program of
the Biological Response Modifiers Program
National Cancer Institute
Frederick Cancer Research Facility
P.O.Box B, Frederick, Maryland 21701
U.S.A.

Motomichi TORISU — The First Dept. of Surgery
Kyushu University School of Medicine
3-1-1 Maidashi, Higashi-ku, Fukuoka 812
Japan

Atsushi UCHIDA — Div. of Immunology, Paterson Laboratories
Christie Hospital and Holt Radium Institute
Manchester M20 9BX
U.K.

Yoh WATANABE — Dept. of Surgery
Kanazawa University School of Medicine
13-1 Takara-machi, Kanazawa 920
Japan

Hiroshi YAMAMOTO — Dept. of Surgery
Saga Medical School
Nabeshima-cho, Saga 840-01
Japan

Etsuro YANAGAWA — Div. of Immunology, Paterson Laboratories
Christie Hospital and Holt Radium Institute
Manchester M20 9BX
U.K.

Takeshi YOSHIDA — Dept. of Pathology
The University of Connecticut Health Center
Framington, Connecticut 06032
U.S.A.

Preface

The Man of Science appears to be the only man who has something to say just now—and the only man who does not know how to say it.
—Sir James Barrie—

During recent years, the basis for adjuvant immunotherapy, single or combined with other therapeutic means, for human cancer is becoming progressively well established. The results of properly designed active immunotherapy with biological response modifiers have proved its effectiveness on the duration of survival for patients with cancer. Especially, OK-432 (Picibanil—a product of Chugai Pharmaceutical Co., Ltd., Japan), a lyophilized powder of the incubation mixture of penicillin-treated low virulent Su-strain of *Streptococcus pyogenes* of human origin, is known to be one of the most useful microbial products of immunotherapeutic agents. Since 1975 when the agent was approved its marketing in Japan and since 1980 when we first reported the clinical results of randomized study of its use for cancer treatment, OK-432 has been widely prescribed in Japan. In addition, in the search for strong biological response modifiers, OK-432 has attracted much attention of many immunologists and oncologists in the countries of Europe and America. Thus, many reports have appeared in medical journals on its biological activities and clinical effectiveness. However, its exact effective mechanisms and pharmacokinetics are not fully understood, and the optimal means of administration is not defined yet.

At the 13th International Congress of Chemotherapy, held in Vienna from August 28 to September 2, 1983, a special session took place entitled "Clinical and Experimental Studies in Immunotherapy" by the organized committee of the congress in order to summarize and discuss the biological activities of this particular agent along with its clinical effectiveness. The session was composed of outstanding international members from Austria, France, Italy, Hungary, Japan, Korea, United Kingdom, U.S.A. and Yugoslavia, who presented remarkable topics of experimental or clinical works on this BRM, OK-432. The main subjects of active discussion during the session included the regulatory and stimulatory mechanisms of OK-432, which control and modulate the immune responses, especially cytotoxic augmentation, and which bring about a prolongation of survival time or at least a reduction of clinical symptoms in the treated cancer patients.

Because of our insufficient immunobiological studies and inadequate accumulation of scientific evidence on this particular agent, we may have had some excessive enthusiasm about the potential of the active immunotherapy of OK-432 in human cancer, but this opportunity was worthwhile for the exchanging of results from past studies, summing up the knowledge so far disclosed and for the exploration of new avenues and strategies for the direction of future programs for both the fundamental and clinical aspects of OK-432, which then certainly will be able to extend to many biological response modifiers in general.

This monograph, which includes all of the papers presented at the session in Vienna, will not only put on record the above mentioned valuable experimental and clinical results of OK-432 studies made by such outstanding scientists and clinicians, but certainly will also stimulate the progress in the field of cancer immunology and immunotherapy.

Finally, I wish to acknowledge all of the members of the Organizing Committee of the 13th International Congress of Chemotherapy for their timely decisions in order to open this session and for their well-arranged management attributed by the success of this session, held in one of the most pleasant and beautiful historical cities with incomparable atmosphere, Vienna.

Takashi Hoshino
Professor of Immunology and Parasitology
Fukui Medical School

CONTENTS

OK-432 (picibanil): Property, action and clinical effectiveness

TAKASHI HOSHINO[1] and ATSUSHI UCHIDA[2]

[1]*Department of Immunology and Parasitology, Fukui Medical School, Fukui, Japan and* [2]*Institute for Applied and Experimental Oncology, University of Wien, Wien, Austria*

Introduction

It has been known for many years that accidental complication with erysipelas (streptococcus hemolyticus infection) often brings about temporal benefits in patients with malignant diseases, suggesting that these particular bacilli have a potential activity against cancer through modification of the host defense mechanisms. Okamoto and his associates,[1] in 1967, discovered a useful preparation of this group of bacilli and designated it as OK-432.

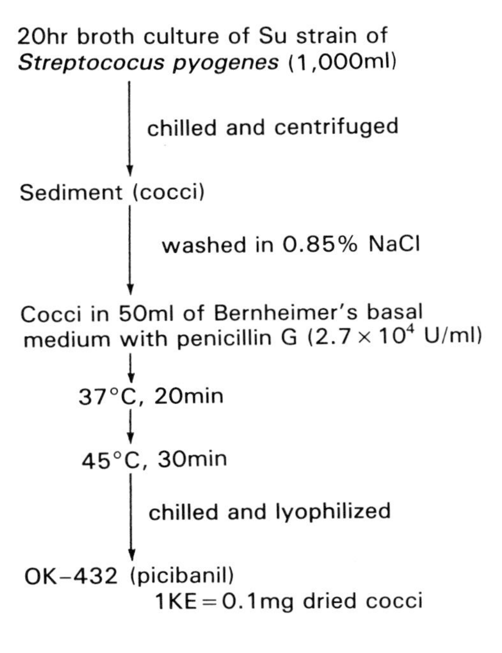

FIGURE 1 *OK-432.*

OK-432 is produced by incubating the low virulent SU strain of *Streptococcus pyogenes* of human origin, treated with penicillin G followed by lyophilization of the incubation mixture (Fig. 1). A unit of KE (Klinische Einheit) is used to express the strength of the preparation, 1 KE corresponding to 0. 1 mg lyophilized bacilli. It is parenterally given through any route, suspended in saline or any other medium. A lack of growing capacity in the bacilli has been confirmed by animal inoculation studies as well as by cultivation in various media following treatment with penicillinase. Since 1975 when OK-432 was given approval for marketing by the Japanese Ministry of Health and Welfare, OK-432 has been widely prescribed to treat cancer patients in Japan and in South Korea. Despite its favorable results, prolonged survival and decreased clinical symptoms of treated patients, its effective mechanisms and the best way of administration are not fully defined yet. My presentation will deal with an overview of the clinical effectiveness and the immunopharmacological functions of OK-432 as a biological response modifier mainly based on the results of our own in vivo and in vitro studies.

Clinical results of OK-432 treatment

In 1980, we first reported the results of a randomized comparative study

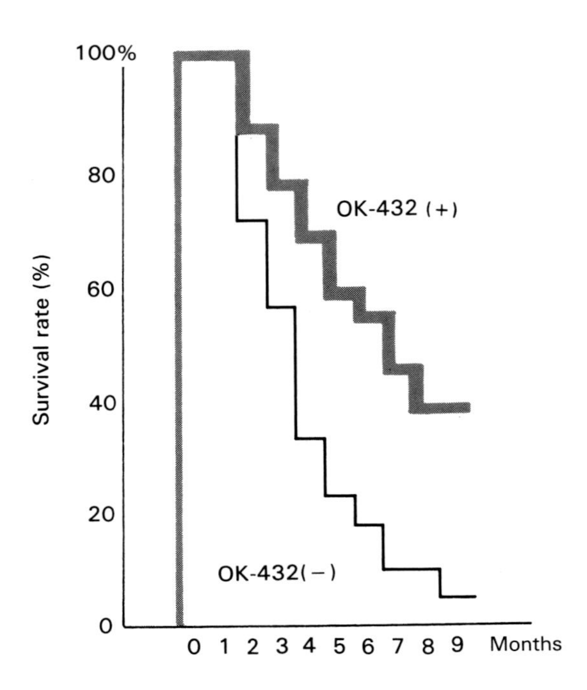

FIGURE 2 *Comparison of survival rate between groups treated with and without OK-432.*

on OK-432 immunotherapy.[2] A series of 44 patients with adenocarcinoma of the stomach and 36 patients with adenocarcinoma of the lung, all of whom were very advanced and in the clinical stages of III or IV, were divided into two groups. The patients in the study group were given OK-432, 5 KE intradermally everyday in combination with 5-FU, while the control group was only given 5-FU. Although most of the patients took a rather downhill course because of the extensive metastasis of the original tumor, the survival rates after the initiation of the therapy were much longer in the patients given 5-FU and OK-432 chemoimmunotherapy than those given chemotherapy with 5-FU alone (Fig. 2). The most conspicuous effect of OK-432 therapy was observed in the 12 months' survival rates, which exceeded 23% in the study group, while all the patients treated with only 5-FU died within 10 months. The results clearly indicate that OK-432 immunotherapy was at least effective for life prolongation even in advanced cancer of the stomach and the lung. The immunological studies performed in the patients given OK-432 showed quantitative and qualitative effectiveness on impaired cell-mediated immunity after the therapy. When the lymphocyte parameters were compared before and 4 weeks after daily intradermal OK-432 injections the OK-432 immunotherapy was proved to produce increased absolute lymphocyte counts above 1,500 per mm^3 and normalization of T cell rate in almost all treated cases. In about half of the treated patients the PHA and Con A blastogenesis increased to within the normal range (Figs. 3 and 4).[2]

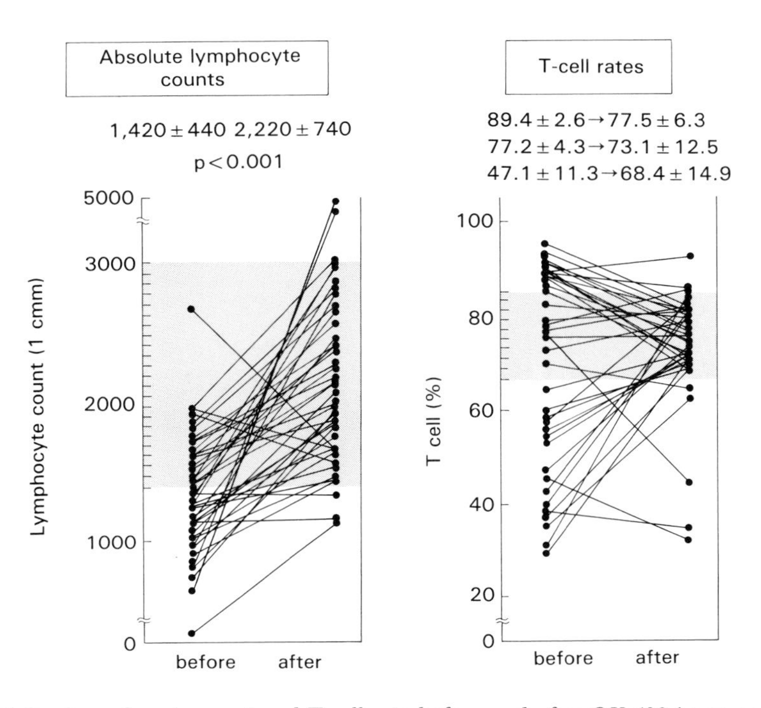

FIGURE 3 *Lymphocyte count and T-cell rate before and after OK-432 immunotherapy.*

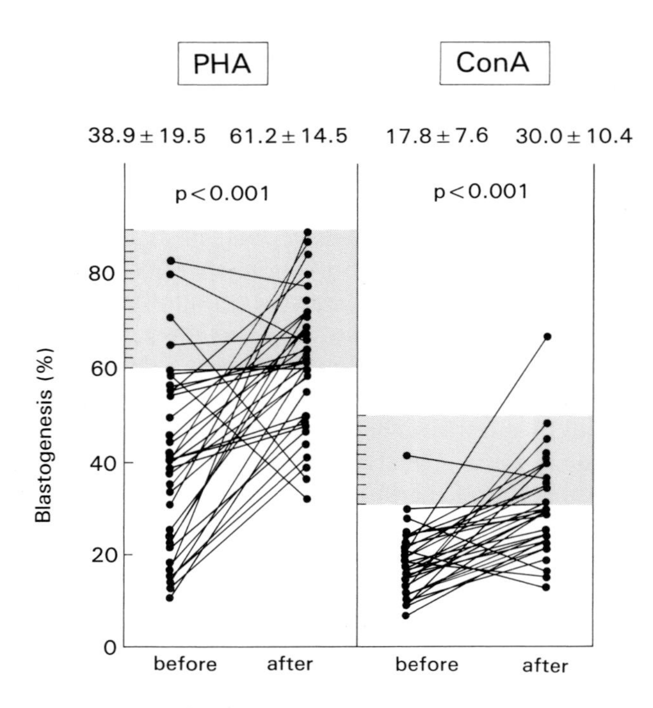

FIGURE 4 *Phytomitogen blastogenic rate of lymphocytes before and after OK-432 immunotherapy.*

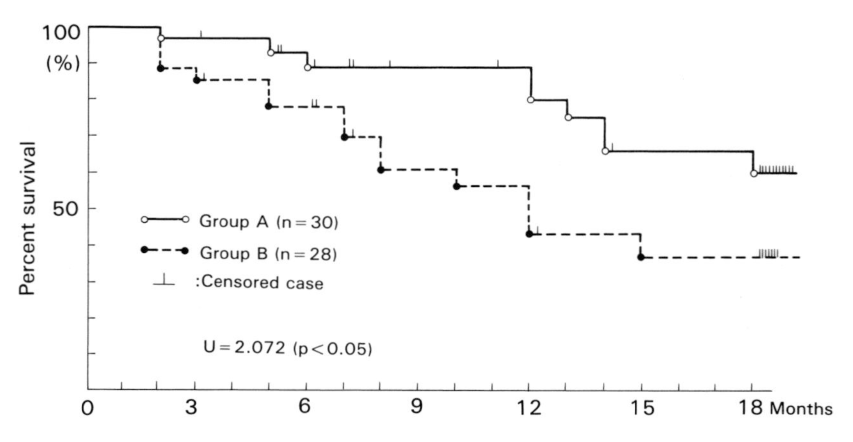

FIGURE 5 *Survival curve of malignant glioma.* (Kaplan-Meier method) (from K. Takakura et al.: 13th International Cancer Congress, Seattle USA, 1982)

Following our report, many clinical experiments were designed and carried out in Japan in order to confirm the clinical effectiveness and to analyze the immunological efficacy of OK-432. Among them, the results of the therapy for carcinomatous pleuritis and peritonitis by Dr. Torisu[3] and the results of a randomized comparative survival study for lung cancer by Dr. Watanabe[4] will be discussed in detail in the later part of the session. I will introduce three more randomized studies recently performed in Japan.

Recent studies of the Brain Tumor Adjuvant Immunotherapy Study Group, conducted by Takakura[5] disclosed the benefits of OK-432 immunotherapy in certain brain tumors. After surgical treatment, patients with malignant glioma were randomized into 2 groups. The 30 patients of group A were given radiotherapy plus ACNU in combination with OK-432, while the 28 patients in group B were given only radiotherapy and ACNU. Both groups were comparable in terms of patients' background, yet a higher survival rate with statistical significance was demonstrated in group A than in group B (Fig. 5).

Shirakawa and his associates[6] reported a favorable remission-prolongating

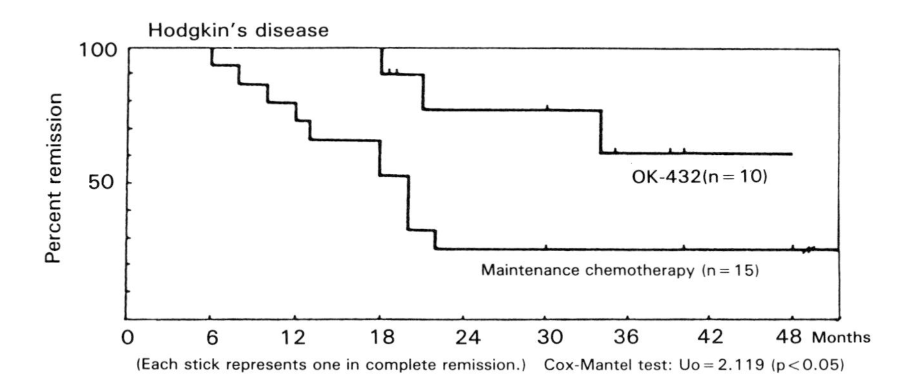

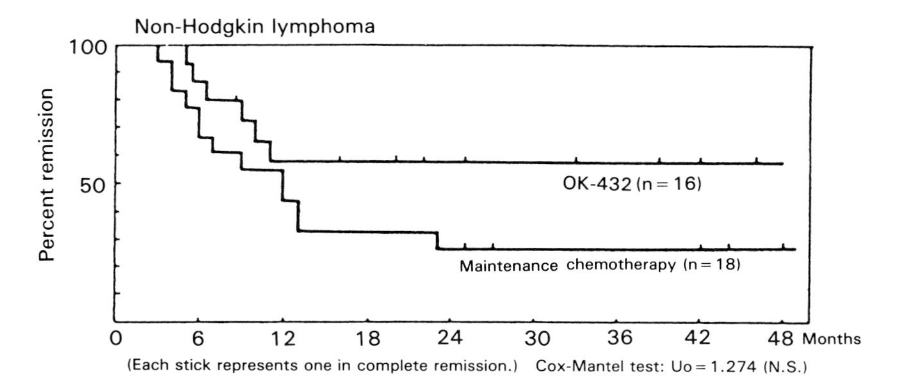

FIGURE 6 *Duration of the complete remission produced by induction chemotherapy in patients with malignant lymphoma. Comparison of two groups given OK-432 alone and maintenance chemotherapy during remission.*
(from S. Shirakawa et al.: 13th International Cancer Congress, Seattle, USA, 1982)

effect from a single treatment of OK-432 rather than of maintenance chemotherapy, in patients with malignant lymphoma. Namely, after the induction of complete remission by a fixed schedule of combination chemotherapy, a total of 55 patients, 25 with Hodgkin's disease and 30 with non-Hodgkin's lymphoma, were randomly divided into 2 groups, one received OK-432 alone and the other received maintenance combined chemotherapy. In both of the Hodgkin's and non-Hodgkin's lymphoma patient groups, the prognosis was significantly better with a decreased relapsing rate and longer duration of remission in the patients given OK-432 alone than those that were treated with chemotherapy during the remission (Fig. 6).

A randomized comparative study on the effect of OK-432 was also carried out by the Japan Cooperative Study Group for Malignant Melanomas, headed by Hayasaka.[7] Among a total of 167 cases of malignant melanoma, 83 (46%) were given chemotherapeutic agents in association with OK-432 and were found to have a survival rate of three years. This rate was significantly higher than that of 20% in 84 cases given chemotherapy alone (Fig. 7).

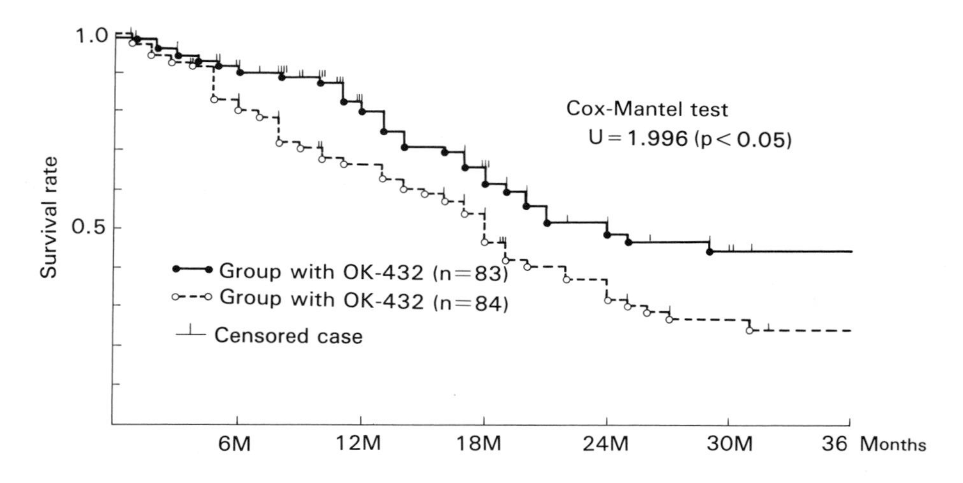

FIGURE 7 *Comparison of the survival curve (all cases with malignant melanoma).* (from K. Hayasaka et al.: 16th International Congress of Dermatology, Tokyo, Japan, 1982)

In summary, it was certainly recognized that OK-432 administration, either alone or in combination with other chemotherapeutic agents, to patients with various types of malignant tumors, successfully prolonged the survival time even in advanced cases. The use of OK-432 was proved to be effective not only in producing a remission together with chemotherapy or radiotherapy but also in the extension of the duration of disease-free remission. Patients successfully treated with OK-432 demonstrated recovery of immune responses to recall antigens in vivo and to increase of mitogenic blastogenesis of lymphocytes in vitro. These data suggest that the mechanisms of action of OK-432 are not directly tumoricidal but seem to operate through activation of the host defense mechanisms. Thus, the effective mechanisms of this preparation, particularly the immunologic functions are of special interest.

Immunological studies on OK-432

So far a number of in vivo and in vitro studies concerning various immunologic functions on OK-432 have been carried out and the results were frequently reported in medical journals of domestic and foreign countries. Therefore, this report will deal only with the effect of OK-432 on NK cell activity of lymphocytes, which has recently been accepted as one of the most important resistances to cancer development and metastasis and has been known to be the most reliable parameter of the action of biological response modifiers.

Augmentation of NK cell activity

Our recent studies[8-10] demonstrated augmentation of NK activity of mononuclear cells (MC) after in vivo injection or in vitro incubation with OK-432 in patients with cancer. The results will be briefly discussed.

(a) NK activity of mononuclear cells in circulating blood (PB-MC) and carcinomatous pleural effusion (PE-MC)

Sixty patients with malignant solid tumors who were off anticancerous drugs and 44 normal men (roughly age-matched) were subjected to the study as experimental and control groups. PB-MC and PE-MC from patients with breast and lung cancer with pleural metastasis showed moderate impairment and marked reduction or even complete absence of NK activity, respectively, compared to that of PB-MC from normal subjects (Fig. 8). A single injection of 5 KE of OK-432 resulted in an increase of NK activity of PB-MC up to 180% of the pretreatment level with the peak in 3 days and a subsequent rapid decrease to the original low levels in 7 days (Fig. 9). The extent of NK augmentation by OK-432 depended on the route of administration. The highest NK augmentation was achieved through intravenous injection, followed by an intradermal route. Since human NK activity is believed to be exerted by large granular lymphocytes (LGL), the time course change of LGL count and rate of LGL-target conjugates were examined, but these values were fairly stationary even after OK-432 administration. Thus the NK enhancing effect of OK-432 might be derived from the enhancement of lytic function of the NK cell.

In order to clarify the effect of OK-432 therapy at the site of the malignant cell proliferation, clinical effectiveness and NK activity of PE-MC was

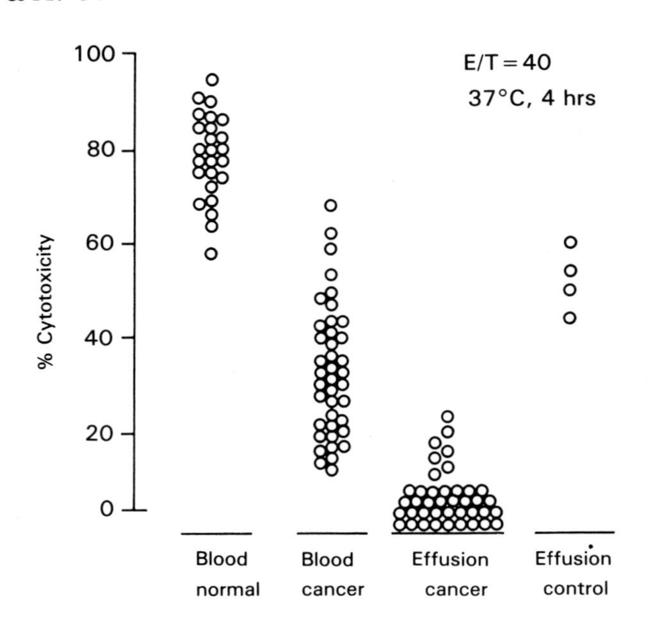

FIGURE 8 *NK activity of mononuclear cells against K562.*

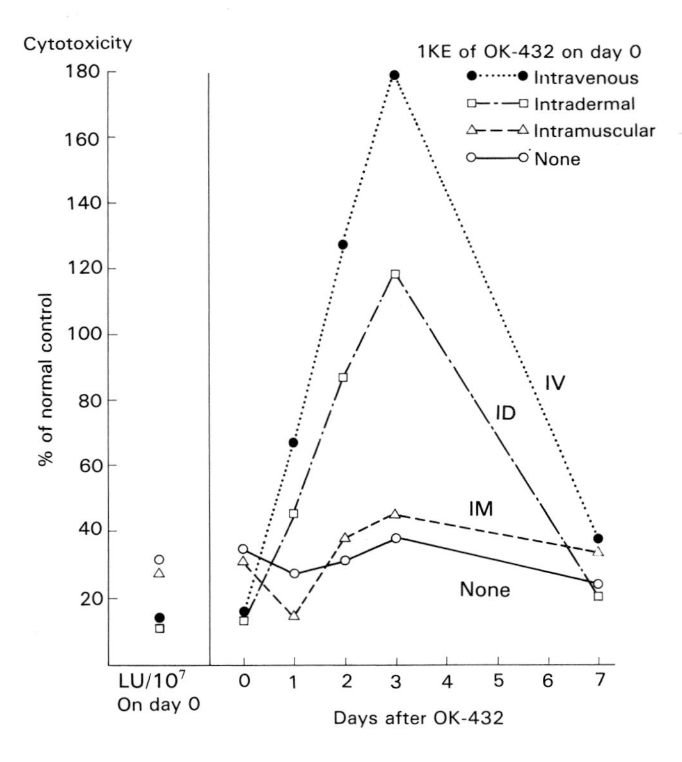

FIGURE 9 *Effect of systemic administration of OK-432 on NK activity.*

traced after intrapleural injection of 10 KE of OK-432 in 12 patients with malignant pleural effusion. Reduction or even disappearance of the effusion was observed in 10 patients (responder), while only 2 cases did not show any effectiveness (non-responder)(Table 1). In addition a marked increase in recovery of NK activity of PE-MC was observed 7 days after the injection in the clinical responder patients, but NK activity remained to be low or absent in 2 non-responder patients (Fig. 10). Thus it is clearly shown that the effectiveness of OK-432 in reducing carcinomatous effusion is achieved through increasing the NK activity. Actually an analysis of cellular composition of PE-MC 7 days after OK-432 therapy disclosed increased

TABLE 1 *Intrapleural administration of OK-432: Clinical effects*

	Effusions	Effusion tumor cells
No change	2/12	2/9
Reduction	7/12	4/9
Disappearance	3/12	3/9

Intrapleural injection of 10KE, OK-432

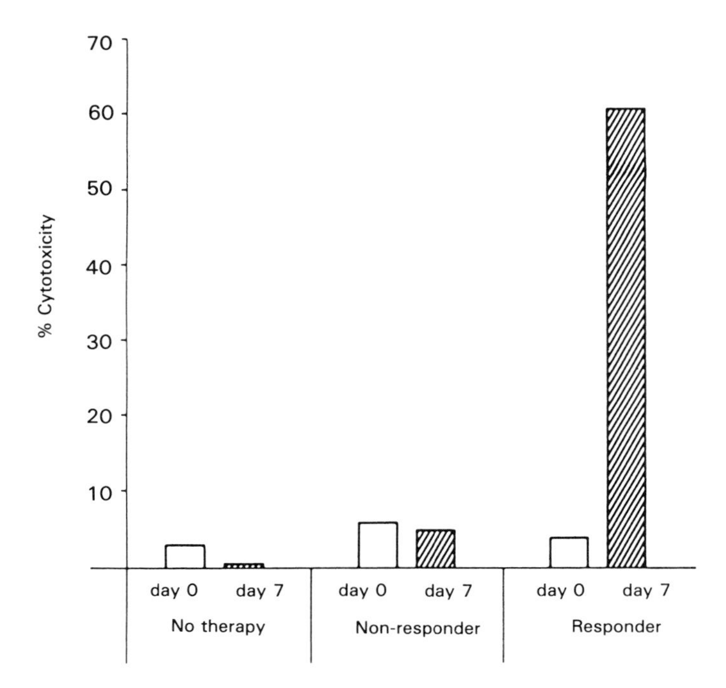

FIGURE 10 *Enhancement of pleural effusion NK cell activity by intrapleural injection of OK-432.*
(OK-432, 10 KE, on day 0) E/T=40

lymphoid cells with decreased tumor cells in responder cases, but no such change of cellular composition was seen in non-responder cases.

(b) Role of macrophage on NK cell activity[11,12]

In searching for the cause of a marked decrease or even absent NK activity in carcinomatous pleural effusion, fractionation of these cells was attempted to look for the responsible components. The frequency of LGL in effusion cells was compatible to that in blood lymphocytes, suggesting that the cause of decreased NK activity is not due to reduced LGL. NK activity of PB-MC from normal men or patient's themselves deteriorated when it was preincubated for 20 hours with macrophages separated from cancer pleural effusion in the dose-response manner (Fig. 11), while Sepadex G-10 column passed and 24 hours' incubated cells showed no such NK suppressing activity to allogeneic normal or autologous circulating lymphocytes. This study confirmed that carcinomatous pleural effusion contains macrophages which are capable of suppressing the development and maintenance of NK activity of lymphocytes. Intrapleural injection of OK-432 resulted in an abrogation of the suppressing activity of these macrophages, and thus the recovery of NK activity of PE-MC was achieved with clinical effect of reduction of effusion (Fig. 12). Similar NK-suppressing macrophage or monocytes were recently discovered by us[13] in the circulating blood of postoperative cancer patients, which may cause the development of metastasis often observed after major surgery for removal of the cancer focus (Fig. 13).

(c) In vitro augmentation of NK activity by OK-432[8]

In vitro incubation of mononuclear cells with OK-432 resulted in the dose of OK-432 and the time of incubation-dependent augmentation of NK activity in both normal subjects and in patients with cancer. The enhancement

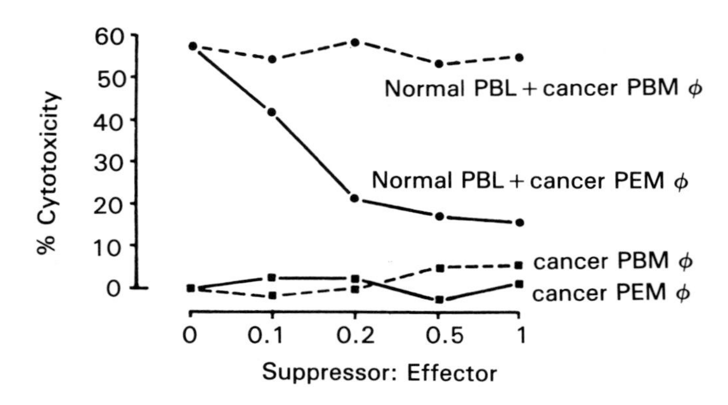

FIGURE 11 *Suppression of NK activity by monocytes.* K562 target E:T = 20:1

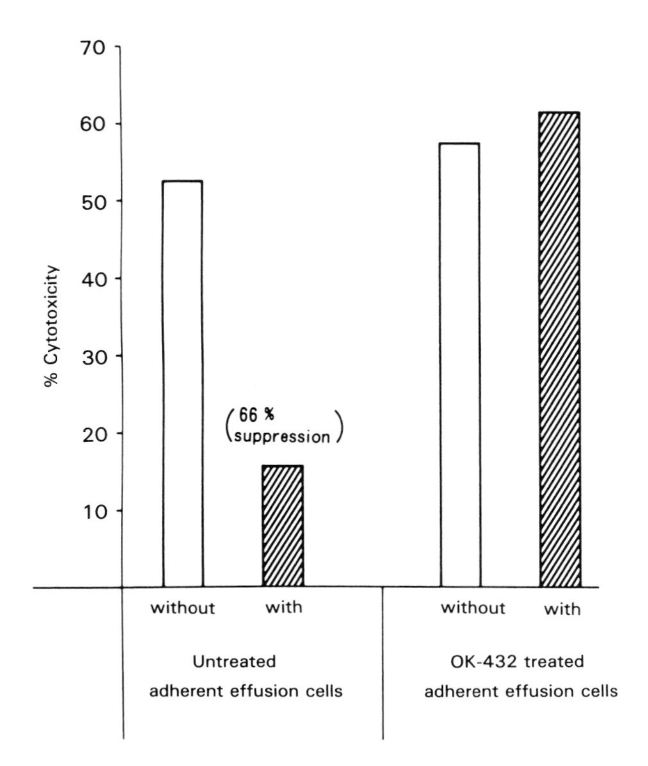

FIGURE 12 *Reduction of NK suppressor cells by intrapleural injection of OK-432.* Blood lymphocytes were cultured for 24 hours with or without adherent effusion cells from patients before and 7 days after the 1st i.p. injection of OK-432. E/T = 40

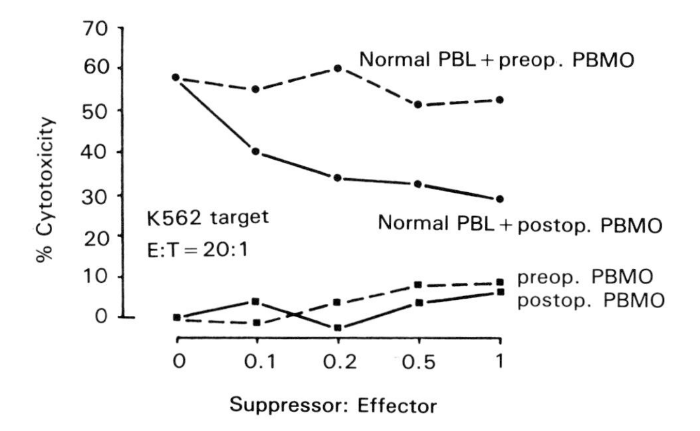

FIGURE 13 *Suppression of NK activity by monocytes from postoperative cancer patients.*

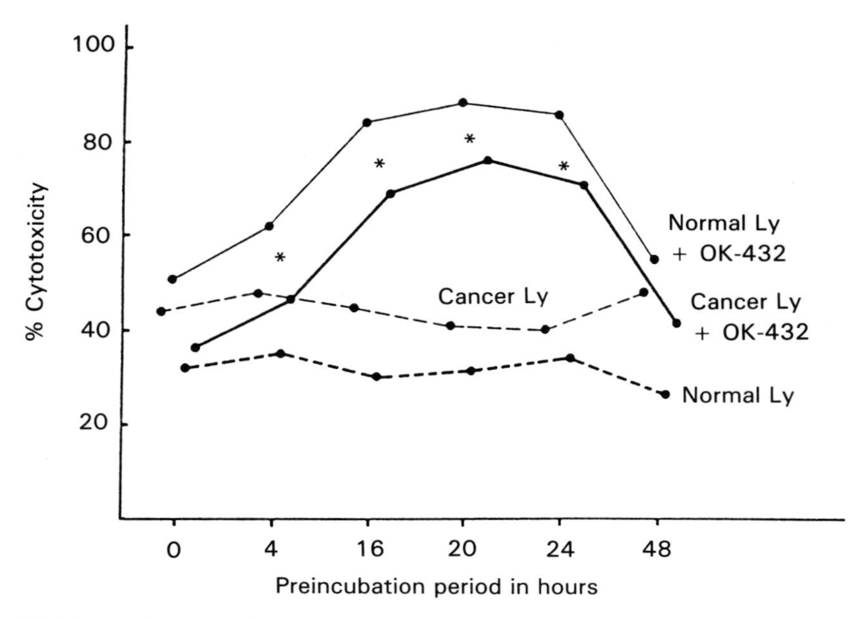

FIGURE 14 *Kinetics of augmentation of cytotoxic activity against K562 cells by OK-432.* Effect of preincubation period. OK-432: 0.5 KE/ml, E/T ratio: 20 (*p<0.05)

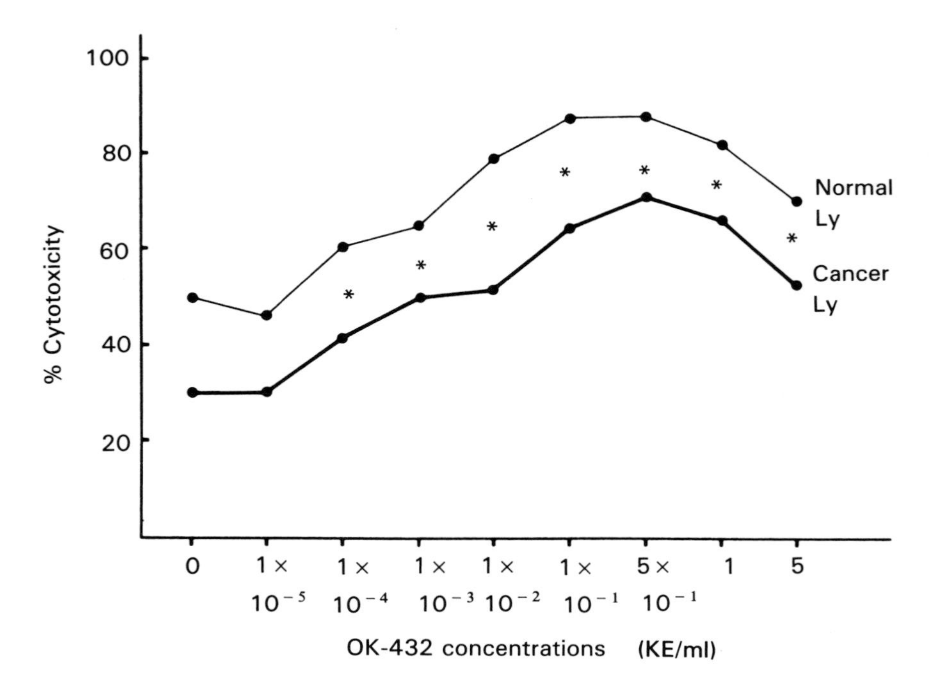

FIGURE 15 *Augmentation of cytotoxic activity against K562 cells by doses of OK-432.* OK-432 incubation for 20 hours, E/T ratio: 20 (*p<0.05)

of NK activity by OK-432 was observed as early as 4 hours of incubation, with the peak effect around 20 hours of incubation (Fig. 14). The mode of intensity of cytotoxic activation of OK-432 was dose dependent with the maximum effect at a concentration of 0.5 KE/ml (Fig. 15). Percoll fractionation study disclosed that the actual augmentation for NK activity is merely performed by the LGL fraction (Fig. 16). Incubation with OK-432 did not alter the rate of LGL and target cell conjugation nor the participation of monocyte or macrophage. Addition of anti-alpha-interferon antibody to the OK-432 incubation mixture did not completely inhibit the boosting activity of OK-432. These results suggest that OK-432 augments the cytotoxic activity of LGL, having the ability to recognize target cells not simply depending on alpha-interferon production.

The mechanism of NK augmentation by OK-432 is one of the most attractive subjects to be investigated. However, since the other reports in this

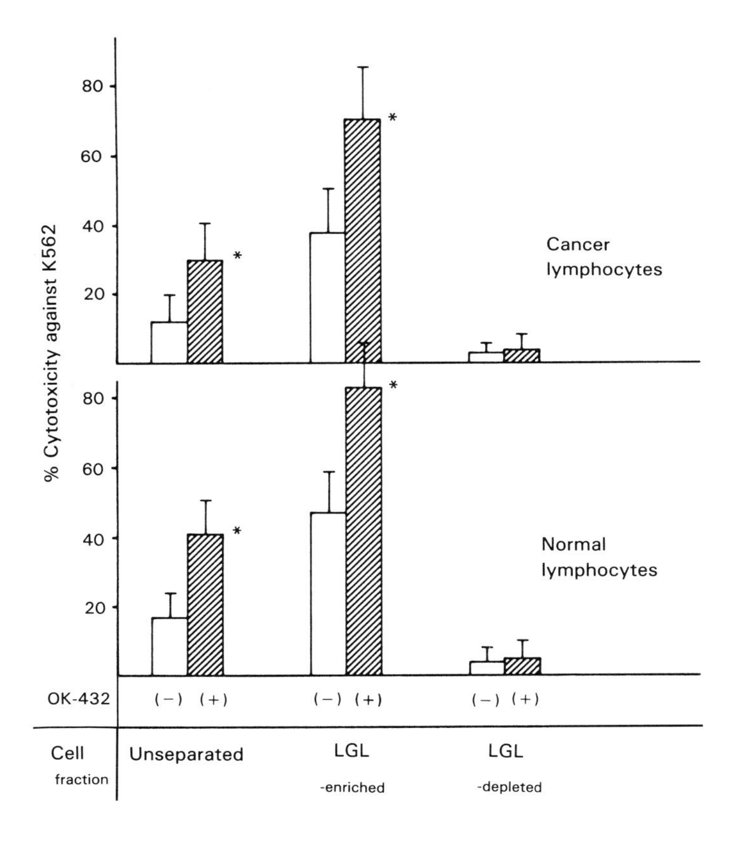

FIGURE 16 *Augmentation of cytotoxic activity of large granular lymphocytes (LGL) by OK-432.*
LGL: collected by Percoll gradient, E/T ratio: 20, No. of cases: 6 in each, *: $p<0.05$

session will contain many different results on these interesting topics, the details about induction of IFN, IL-2, IL-1 and other lymphokines by OK-432 stimulation will not be discussed here.[14-16] However, it should be emphasized that OK-432 is not a simple inducer of these humoral factors, but seems to produce a certain specific cytotoxic or regulatory humoral factor(s).

Augmentation of autologous cytotoxicity by OK-432[17-20]

It is well known that NK cells are hard to kill their own fresh tumor cells. In order to search whether or not the augmented NK activity induced by stimulation with OK-432 is capable of killing own tumor cells in or around the original and metastatic sites, autologous cytotoxicity was examined against the tumor cells separated from pleural effusion. PB-MC incubated with OK-432 definitely showed a higher rate of lymphocyte cytotoxicity against ^{51}Cr-labeled own fresh tumor cells than that unstimulated by PB-MC or stimulated with IFN-α (Fig. 17). When an individual case is analyzed, circulating lymphocytes in 4 out of 5 cases displayed OK-432 induced autologous cytotoxicity by 24 hrs' incubation (Table 2). Effusion mononuclear cells also showed similar or higher OK-432 induced autologous cytotoxicity (Table 3). On the other hand, IFN-α failed to produce or to modulate the autologous cytotoxicity. In fact, intrapleural injection of OK-432 in patients with carcinomatous pleural effusion resulted in a definite augmentation of autologous cytotoxicity of PE-MC in so-called responded cases but not in non-responded cases (Table 4). A similar augmentation of autologous cytotoxicity was also observed against lymphoma cells of extripated lymph node by PB-MC preincubated with OK-432 for 16 hours, but not with IFN-α or IL-2 in patients with malignant lymphoma (Table 5).

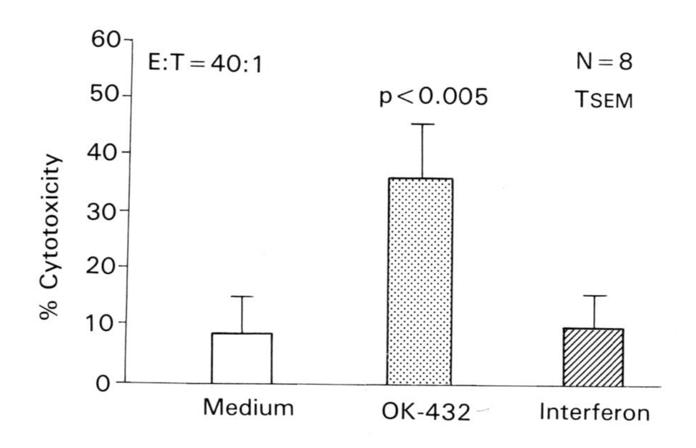

FIGURE 17 *OK-432–induced autologous lymphocytotoxicity.*

TABLE 2 *Blood autologous lymphocytotoxicity: OK-432, interferon*

Exp.	% Cytotoxicity at E:T of 80:1		
	Medium	OK-432	IFN
1	0	16[a]	−2
2	5	29[a]	0
3	21	33[a]	19
4	−4	11[a]	3
5	4	−3	7

a) $p < 0.05$

TABLE 3 *Effusion autologous lymphocytotoxicity: OK-432, interferon*

Exp.	% Cytotoxicity at E:T of 80:1		
	Medium	OK-432	IFN
1	0	12[a]	3
2	4	57[a]	2
3	−3	14[a]	−5
4	25	39[a]	29
5	7	−2	0

a) $p < 0.05$

TABLE 4 *Effusion autologous lymphocytotoxicity: Induction by intrapleural OK-432 injection*

OK-432 treatment[a]	% Cytotoxicity	
	Day 0	Day 7
None	2 (0–7)	3 (0–6)
Non-responder	1 (0–2)	3 (0–6)
Responder[b]	3 (0–10)	29 (7–75)[c]

a) I. pl. injection of 10KE OK-432 on day 0.
b) Reduction of effusion tumor cells.
c) $p < 0.05$

TABLE 5 *Effect of in vitro treatment of effector cells with OK-432 on lymphocyte cytotoxicity against autologous lymph node cells and K562 (NK)*

E/T = 25

Case #	Histological diagnosis	Effector cell	% Cytotoxicity of PB-MN from patient				% Cytotoxicity of PB-MN from normal subject			
		Pretreatment	(−)	OK-432	(−)	OK-432	(−)	OK-432	(−)	OK-432
		target cell	Autologous LN cells		K562		Patient's LN cell		K562	
12	Diffuse med. sized		0	8.2	10.3	51.1	9.8	4.1	36.2	57.2
13	〃 〃		15.0	9.3	4.0	14.1	12.3	26.5	N.D.	N.D.
14	〃 large call		2.7	17.1	9.8	22.1	10.7	15.8	16.4	37.0
15	〃 〃		0	0	8.2	8.8	0	N.D.	25.3	N.D.
17	〃 small cell		0	11.1	69.0	78.5	0	5.6	12.7	25.1
18	Follicular med. sized		4.3[a]	22.6[a]	31.0[a]	66.6[a]	4.0[a]	6.3[a]	25.2[a]	37.4[a]
19	Hodgkin's disease		1.2	3.1	2.5	1.4	N.D.	N.D.	N.D.	N.D.
20	IBL or ch. lymphadenitis		0	2.9	17.2	26.5	0	9.8	35.5	43.6
21	Ch. lymphadenitis		0	4.1	12.1	33.3	0	5.6	24.5	72.7

a) E/T = 50

Other immunologic functions of OK-432

Other than those described above, OK-432 is known to have many other important immunologic functions, such as an adjuvant effect when combined with lectin or vaccine, activation of complement system in serum and on the surface of malignant cells, increases of endogenous and exogenous hematopoietic stimulating factors and neutrophil-mediated tumor cell destruction in OK-432 injected cancerous ascites along with an evidence of cytostatic effect on neutrophils. It is certain that many other actions of OK-432 which modify biological functions will be clarified accompanying the progress of immunological procedures.

Conclusions

Immunotherapy with OK-432 was discussed in both the clinical and experimental viewpoints. Administration of OK-432 either alone or in combination with chemotherapy or radiotherapy has been confirmed to at least be effective in prolonging the survival of patients with cancer, even in advanced stages. Patients successfully treated with OK-432 clearly showed recovery from impaired immune response, especially in cell mediated immunity, suggesting the mechanism of action of OK-432 is by the activation of the immune defense system. In vivo and in vitro immunological studies in human and animal demonstrated multiple and complicated functions of OK-432 including activation of T cell mediated cytotoxicity, modulation of regulatory T cells, activation of cytotoxic or cytostatic macrophage through increased target binding and phagocytosis, augmentation of NK cell activity in accordance with production of IFN-γ, IL-1, IL-2, elimination or impotency of NK suppressor macrophage and probably other additional NK enhancing factors and finally the augmentation of autologous cytotoxicity. Although clinical indications and the best means of administration of OK-432 are not conclusively defined yet, and there still are many additional studies to be performed to clarify the effective mechanisms of OK-432, the preparation is believed to be hopeful and a useful tool for the treatment of malignant diseases.

References

1. Okamoto, H., Minami, M. and Shoin, S. (1966): Experimental anticancer studies part XXXI. On the streptococcal preparation having potent anticancer activity. *Jpn. J. Exp. Med., 36,* 175.
2. Uchida, A. and Hoshino, T. (1980): Clinical studies on cell-mediated immunity in patients with malignant disease. I. Effect of immunotherapy with OK-432 on lymphocyte subpopulation and phytomitogen responsiveness in vitro. *Cancer, 45,* 476.

3. Torisu, M., Katano, M., Kimura, Y., Itoh, H. and Takesue, M. (1983): Approach to management of malignant ascites with a streptococcal preparation, OK-432. I. Improvement of host immunity and prolongation of survival. *Surgery, 93,* 357.
4. Watanabe, Y. and Iwa, T. (1982): Results of immunotherapy by streptococcal preparation, OK-432, as an adjuvant for resected lung cancer. In: *Proceed. 13th Intern. Congress of Cancer,* pp. 358. Editors: E.A. Mirand, W.B. Hutchinson and E. Mihich. Liss, New York.
5. Takakura, K. (1982): Effects of adjuvant immunotherapy with OK-432 on malignant glioma. In: *Proceed. 13th Intern. Congress of Cancer,* pp. 165. Editors: E.A. Mirand, W.B. Hutchinson and E. Mihich. Liss, New York.
6. Shirakawa, S., Karitani, R., Nishigori, S., Fukuhara, S., Nasu, K., Kita, K. and Uchino, A. (1982): Remission maintenance immunotherapy by OK-432, A streptococcus pyogenes preparation, in malignant lymphoma. In: *Proceed. 13th Intern. Congress of Cancer,* pp. 412. Editors: E.A. Mirand, W.B. Hutchinson and E. Mihich. Liss, New York.
7. Hayasaka, K. (1982): Immunochemotherapy of malignant melanoma by Picibanil. In: *Proceed. 16th Intern. Congress of Dermatol.,* Tokyo.
8. Uchida, A. and Micksche, M. (1981): In vitro augmentation of natural killing activity by OK-432. *Intern. J. Immunophar., 3,* 365.
9. Uchida, A., Micksche, M. and Hoshino T. (1982): Effect of OK-432 on the natural killer activity of mononuclear cells in circulating blood and carcinomatous pleural effusion. In: *Immunomodulation by Microbial Products and Related Synthetic Compounds,* pp. 446. Editors: Y. Yamamura et al., Excerpta Medica, Amsterdam.
10. Uchida, A. and Micksche, M. (1982): Augmentation of human natural killing activity by OK-432. In: *NK cells and other natural effector cells,* pp. 431. Editors: R.B. Herberman et al., Academic Press, New York.
11. Uchida, A. and Micksche, M. (1982): Augmentation of NK cell activity in cancer patients by OK-432: Activation of NK cells and reduction of suppressor cells. In: *NK cells and other natural effector cells.* pp. 1303. Editors: R.B. Herberman et al., Academic Press, New York.
12. Uchida, A. and Micksche, M. (1981): Suppressor cells for natural killer activity in carcinomatous pleural effusions of cancer patients. *Cancer Immunol. Immunother., 11,* 255.
13. Uchida, A. Kolb, R. and Micksche, M. (1982): Generation of suppressor cells for natural killer activity in cancer patients after surgery. *J. Nat. Cancer Inst., 68,* 735.
14. Wakasugi, H., Oshimi, K., Miyata, M. and Morioka, Y. (1981): Augmentation of natural killer (NK) cell activity by a streptococcal preparation, OK-432, in patients with malignant tumors. *J. Clin. Immunol., 1,* 154.
15. Oshimi, K., Wakasugi, H., Seki, H. and Kano, S. (1980): Streptococcal preparation OK-432 augments cytotoxic activity against an erythroleukemic cell-line in humans. *Cancer Immunol. Immunother., 9,* 187.
16. Saito, M., Ebina, T., Koi, M., Yamaguchi, T., Kawade, Y. and Ishida, N. (1982): Induction of interferon-gamma in mouse spleen cells by OK-432, a preparation of Streptococcus pyogenes. *Cellular Immunol., 68,* 187.
17. Uchida, A. and Micksche, M. (1982): Autologous mixed lymphocyte reaction in the peripheral blood and pleural effusions of cancer patients. *J. Clin. Invest., 70,* 98.
18. Uchida, A. and Micksche, M. (1983): Lysis of fresh human-tumor cells by autologous large granular lymphocytes from peripheral blood and pleural effusions. *Intern. J. Cancer, 32,* 37.
19. Uchida, A. and Micksche, M. (1983): Lysis of fresh human tumor cells by autologous peripheral blood lymphocytes and pleural effusion lymphocytes activated by OK-432.

J. Nat. Cancer Inst., 71, 673.

20. Yagita, M., Sugiyama, H. and Hoshino, T. (1983): Cytotoxic activity of peripheral blood mononuclear cells (PBMN) against autologous lymphoma cells and allogenic tumor cell lines (K-562) in patients with malignant lymphoma. *Jpn. J. Clin. Hemat., 24,* 368.

The immunomodulatory activity of picibanil (OK-432)*

MICHAEL A. CHIRIGOS[1], TOHRU SAITO[1] and JAMES E. TALMADGE[2]

[1]*Immunopharmacology Section, Biological Therapeutics Branch, Biological Response Modifiers Program, Division of Cancer Treatment, and* [2]*Preclinical Screening Program of the Biological Response Modifiers Program, National Cancer Institute-Frederick Cancer Research Facility, Frederick, MD, U.S.A.*

OK-432, a pharmaceutical preparation of a low virulent Su strain of *Streptococcus pyogenes* developed in Japan,[1] has been reported to possess immunomodulatory activity in preclinical and clinical studies.[2,3] We examined OK-432 in several in vitro and in vivo assays to test its effect on cellular effector cells (natural killer cells, NK; macrophages, Mϕ; cytotoxic T lymphocytes, CTL) against various tumor target cells, and its capacity to act as an adjuvant to tumor cell vaccines.

Employing the assay described for measuring NK cell augmentation,[4] we tested various concentrations of OK-432 for its in vitro capacity to augment splenic NK cell cytotoxicity (Fig. 1). Significant augmentation of NK cytotoxicity occurred with 0.001 μg/ml, with peak activity occurring at 1 μg/ml and declining at higher concentrations. The response to 1 μg/ml approached that achieved with γIFN or poly I:C. OK-432 was tested for its capacity to activate Mϕ directly in vitro to exert tumoricidal activity on P815 radiolabeled target cells (Fig. 2). Levels of OK-432 beginning with 0.1 μg/ml directly activated Mϕ. Peak activation was attained with 50 μg/ml, and was similar to the Mϕ activation achieved by two other known Mϕ activators, poly ICLC and lipopolysaccharide (LPS).

Different responses in augmentation of NK cells were seen depending upon the route by which OK-432 was administered (Table 1). When the intravenous (i.v.) route was used, significant increases in NK cell augmentation occurred only in the spleen and peripheral blood. The highest response occurred at the 4 to 6 mg/kg doses. In contrast, intraperitoneal (i.p.) treat-

* This project has been funded at least in part with Federal funds from the Department of Health and Human Services, under contract number NO1-CO-23910 with Program Resources, Inc. The contents of this publication do not necessarily reflect the views or policies of the Department of Health and Human Services, nor does mention of trade names, commercial products, or organizations imply endorsement by the U.S. Government.

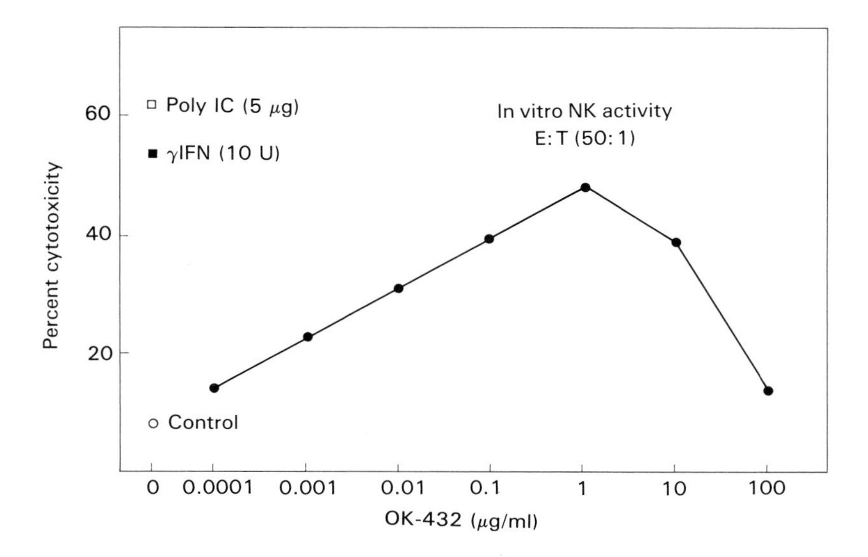

FIGURE 1 *NK cell activity to various doses of OK-432 in vitro.*
Spleens from normal C3H mice were titrated and prepared as a single cell suspension and incubated in the presence of increasing concentrations of OK-432 or polyinosinic polycytidylic acid (poly IC) or murine γ interferon (γIFN) for 20 hr at 37°C in a humidified 5% CO_2-in-air incubator. The cells were washed free of drugs and an effector (spleen cells) to target cell (YAC) ratio of 50:1 incubated for 4 hr to measure cytotoxicity.

TABLE 1 *NK cell augmentation in various compartments to various doses of OK-432 administered by the intravenous or intraperitoneal route*

OK-432 mg/kg[a]	Percent cytotoxicity[b]				
	Intravenous			Intraperitoneal	
	Spleen 50:1	Blood 6:1	TPEC 50:1	Spleen 50:1	TPEC 50:1
Placebo	10	1	4	10	6
0.5	17	7	3	12	36
1.0	23	12	4	10	57
2.0	24	17	5	11	58
4.0	33	21	4	10	56
6.0	30	25	3	9	55
8.0	25	22	4	10	57

a) Mice injected i.v. or i.p. and sacrificed 3 days later for assay.
b) Effector to target ratio of spleen (total cell population); blood (Ficoll-Hypaque separated lymphocytes); TPEC (total peritoneal exudate cells): YAC target cells.

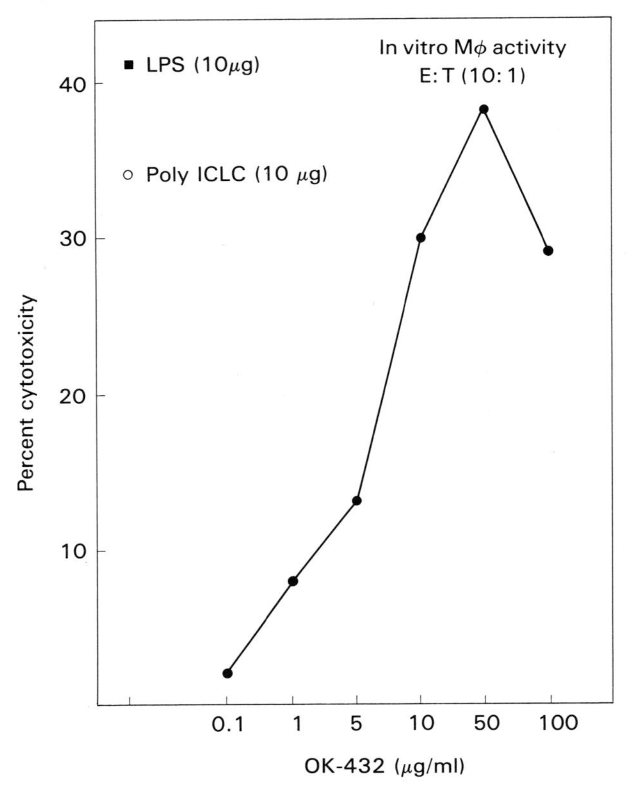

FIGURE 2 *Macrophage activity to various doses of OK-432 in vitro.* Thioglycollate-elicited macrophages from C57BL/6 mice were collected by peritoneum lavage, washed, and allowed to adhere for 4 hr. The effector (Mϕ) to target (^{111}In-labeled P815 tumor cells) ratio of 10:1 was used. Poly ICLC and lipopolysaccharide (LPS) were employed as internal controls. The 72-hr assay was used to measure cytotoxicity (Norbury and Fidler, 1975).[5]

TABLE 2 *Duration of NK cell augmentation following OK-432 treatment*

Route	NK cell source	Day of observation[a)]							
		1	2	3	4	7	9	10	P1[c)]
i.v.	Spleen[b)]	43	65	60	56	33	24		18
i.p.	Spleen[b)]	5		6		8		10	6
	TPEC[b)]	20		61		60		58	5

a) Percent cytotoxicity on indicated day of sacrifice following treatment with 4 mg/kg.
b) Effector to target ratio of 50:1.
c) Placebo-treated control.

ment resulted in significant augmentation of peritoneal NK cell activity without significant splenic NK cell response. Peak total peritoneal exudate cell (TPEC) NK activity occurred at the 1.0 mg/kg dose without a further increase in response at the higher doses.

Based on the results of the dose response studies (Table 1), the 4 mg/kg dose was selected to examine the duration of time that NK cell activity remained elevated following one injection by either the i.p. or i.v. route (Table 2). Splenic NK activity was significantly elevated one day following treatment and remained elevated for seven days, with the peak occurring by the second or third day. As previously observed (Table 1), no significant elevation occurred in the spleen of mice injected by the i.p. route. NK cell activity was augmented within the first day, reaching peak level by the third day and remaining elevated during the ten-day observation period.

To further confirm that variations in NK cell response in various compartments is dependent upon the route by which OK-432 is administered, studies were conducted to compare NK cell response in the three compartments in mice administered 4 mg/kg of OK-432 (Fig. 3). Animals were

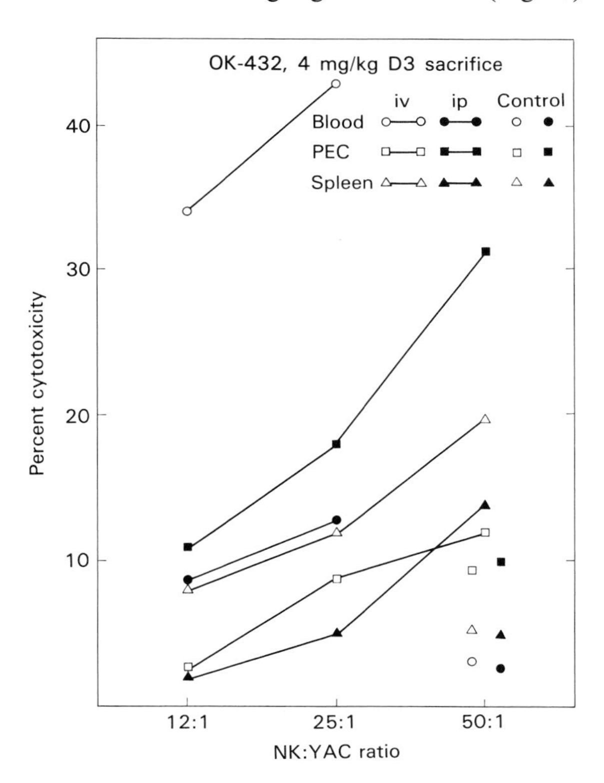

FIGURE 3 *Responses of NK cells in spleen, blood and peritoneum following OK-432 treatment.*

Mice were injected with 4 mg/kg of OK-432 by the i.v. or i.p. route and sacrificed 3 days following treatment.

sacrificed three days following treatment, the time which was shown to be the peak time of NK cell response. The results confirm the previous observations that i.v. treatment results in elevated NK cell cytotoxic activity in blood and spleen but not in total peritoneal exudate cells (PEC). Considering the low effector to target cell ratios used (12:1, 25:1), a very significant response was attained in blood. In contrast, OK-432 administration by the i.p. route resulted in significant NK cell augmentation only in PEC.

It was important to determine whether the level of NK cell activity would be altered as the result of multiple treatments with OK-432. Previous studies with MVE-2 show that multiple treatments with this agent result in a depression of splenic NK cell activity indicating the development of a hyporesponsiveness to the drug.[6] Results in Table 3 show that multiple treatments with OK-432 result in a depression of activity compared to the response attained with one treatment. However, the depression was not as drastic as that resulting from multiple treatments with MVE-2, where NK levels were the same as the placebo-treated controls. The response of TPEC NK cell activity did not appear to be altered by the multiple treatments with either OK-432 or MVE-2.

Various immunomodulating agents have been reported to stimulate the production and secretion of colony stimulating factor (CSF) as reported for Azimexone[7] and for Bacillus Calmette-Guérin.[8] The serum of mice treated with OK-432 was examined for the presence of CSF (Fig. 4). Significant increases in CSF were found in the serum of mice treated with 4 mg/kg. No end point titration was examined above the 4 mg/kg dose. Using a dose of 4 mg/kg, which gave the highest serum content of CSF, we examined the time of appearance of CSF and the duration of time it remained elevated. Peak serum levels appeared on the third day after treatment and slowly declined by the eighth day, although significant levels were still present at that time period.

TABLE 3 *NK cell response to single vs. multiple treatment with OK-432 or MVE-2*

Route	NK cell source	No. of treatments	Percent cytotoxicity[a)]					
			OK-432 (4 mg/kg)			MVE-2 (25 mg/kg)		
			50:1	25:1	12:1	50:1	25:1	12:1
i.v.	Spleen[b)]	1	35	34	25	38	31	20
i.v.	Spleen[b)]	8	21	14	8	2	0	0
i.p.	TPEC[b)]	1	41	33	23	49	32	27
i.p.	TPEC[b)]	3	49	39	27	54	37	23

a) Placebo-treated control values have been subtracted from experimental values.
b) Mice received indicated number of daily treatments and were sacrificed 3 days following the last treatment for NK cell assay.

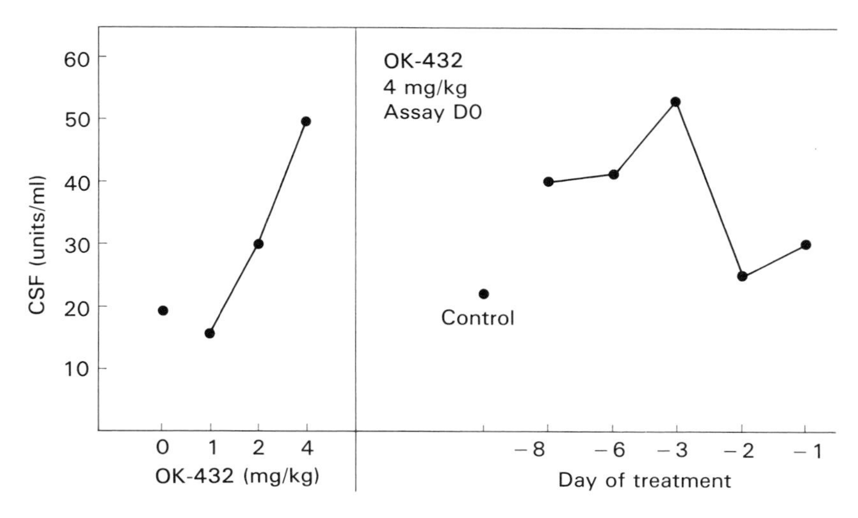

FIGURE 4 *Induction of colony stimulating factor following OK-432 treatment.* Mice were injected with various doses of OK-432 (left panel) or at different time intervals (days) with 4 mg/kg OK-432 (right panel) and sacrificed for serum. CSF is expressed in units/ml, calculated from the number of myeloid colonies formed by 10^5 bone marrow cells in the presence of 1.0 ml of the CSF source.

OK-432 was also examined to assess its capacity to stimulate cytotoxic T-lymphocyte response in an allogeneic tumor system employing the techniques previously reported.[9,10] The results in Table 4 show that OK-432 admixed with the allogeneic tumor cells significantly augmented the cytotoxic T-lymphocyte response to the tumor antigen. A similar adjuvant effect was observed when OK-432 was mixed with UV2237 fibrosarcoma tumor vaccine and syngeneic mice challenged with viable tumor cells (Table 5). Significant protection was attained when OK-432 was mixed with the irradiated tumor cells. At the 20 and 2 μg doses, significant protection occurred against the syngeneic tumor challenge in both parameters: the percent of animals which did not develop tumors, and the rate of growth of the tumor in animals which developed tumors. These results are in keeping with a T-lymphocyte response, and are indicative of the capacity of OK-432 to stimulate the T-cell compartment of the immune system.

B16 melanoma cells, when injected i.v., lodge in the lungs and grow out into macroscopic colonies of tumor. Proliferation is progressive and the number of countable tumor colonies increase with time, leading to eventual death of the animal. We tested the prophylactic effect of OK-432 in this system to assess whether NK cells and/or Mϕ in the lung would prevent establishment of B16 tumor colonies (Table 6). Treatment with 0.5 or 5.0 mg/kg two days prior to challenge with B16 melanoma tumor cells resulted

TABLE 4 *OK-432 adjuvant effect on cytotoxic T-lymphocyte response*

OK-432 total dose[a)]	Tumor vaccine[b)]	Percent cytotoxicity[c)]		
		200:1	100:1	50:1
Placebo (HBSS)	−	15	13	12
Placebo (HBSS)	+	13	15	11
100 μg	−	13	11	11
10 μg	−	13	10	8
1 μg	−	12	9	8
100 μg	+	42	31	19
10 μg	+	28	20	13
1 μg	+	19	13	10

a) OK-432 mixed with irradiated (10,000 R) tumor cell vaccine at time of intradermal injection.
b) Irradiated tumor cells (fibrosarcoma UV2237) injected on day 0 (5×10^6 cells, primary) and day 10 (2×10^6 cells, secondary).
c) On day 15, nonadherent spleen cells were incubated with the radiolabeled (^{75}Se-selenium methionine) clone 46 subline (clonal subline of fibrosarcoma UV2237) at the spleen cell to tumor cell target ratios shown.

TABLE 5 *OK-432 adjuvant effect with tumor cell vaccine*

OK-432 total dose[a)]	Tumor vaccine[b)]	% with tumor (average size cm^3)[c)]	
		day 18	day 35
Placebo	−	100 (0.15)	100 (1.90)
Placebo	+	80 (0.21)	80 (1.17)
20 μg	−	100 (0.15)	100 (1.73)
2 μg	−	100 (0.12)	100 (1.71)
0.2 μg	−	100 (0.12)	100 (1.96)
20 μg	+	40 (0.05)	60 (0.33)
2 μg	+	40 (0.10)	40 (1.20)
0.2 μg	+	100 (0.10)	100 (2.10)

a) OK-432 mixed with irradiated (10,000 R) 10^6 UV2237 tumor cell vaccine at time of intradermal injection (i.d.).
b) Tumor cell vaccine injected i.d. on day −10 and viable UV2237 (2×10^5) injected i.d. on day 0.
c) Average size of tumor of animals with tumor.

in significant protection. The 5 mg/kg dose was as effective as poly I:C, our internal positive control standard employed in this assay. A second tumor assay system was used to determine whether activation of NK cells and/or Mφ in the peritoneum would protect against a challenge of lymphoma ascites tumor cells (Fig. 5). The most significant protective effect occurred when OK-432 was administered three days prior to tumor cell challenge. Treatment at this time resulted in the highest increase in survival

TABLE 6 *Antitumor prophylactic effect of OK-432*

Drug	Dose mg/kg	Lung tumors median
HBSS	Placebo	245
OK-432	5	18
OK-432	0.5	118
OK-432	0.05	195
OK-432	0.005	300
Poly I:C	0.5	22

Mice treated with drug i.v. at 2 days prior to B16 melanoma inoculation (5×10^4, i.v.). Mice sacrificed 3 weeks after tumor cell injection for lung tumor counts.

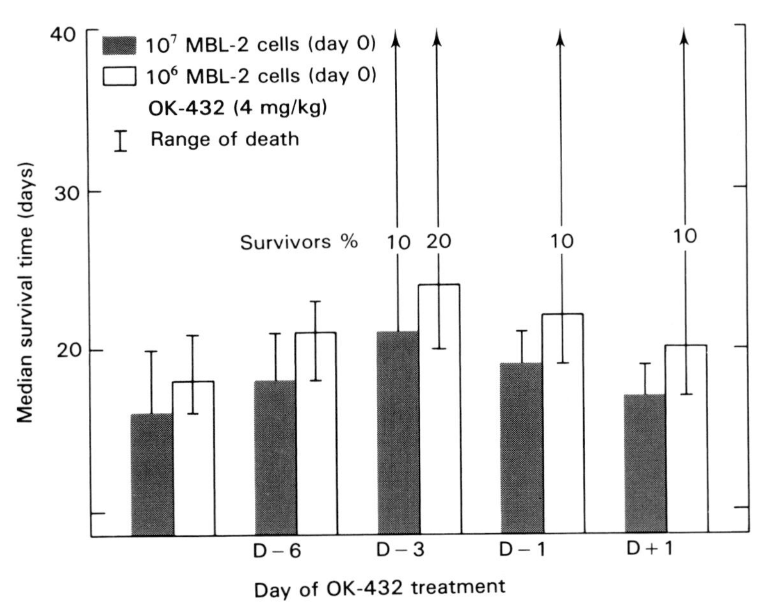

FIGURE 5 *Prophylactic antitumor effect of OK-432.*
C57BL/6 mice were treated i. p. on the indicated days, prior to or after i. p. inoculation of tumor cells (day O).

time as well as in a significant number of long-term survivors. Based on the previous studies which show that the peak of NK and Mϕ response occurs three days after OK-432 treatment, the results (Fig. 5) indicate that the increase in MST was due to a decrease in the number of tumor cells resulting from NK cell and/or Mø tumor cell cytotoxicity.

The last study (Table 7) shows the results of combining cyto-reductive treatment with OK-432. An additive therapeutic response was achieved when the combination was employed to decrease the number of liver and lung tumors and to increase the survival times (groups 5 vs. 6 and group 7 vs. 8 and 9). The observation that Cytoxan pretreatment (group 2) resulted in an increase in the number of liver and lung tumors indicates the immunosuppressive effect of Cytoxan on NK or Mø response in the liver and lung. This also led to the earlier death of this group. The decrease in liver and lung lesions resulting from early Cytoxan treatment, as well as the increase in survival time (group 4 vs. 1), reflects a better therapeutic response due to a lower tumor burden being present four days after tumor cell inoculation, in contrast to treatment on day 7 (group 4 vs. 5). Treatment with OK-432 alone (group 10 and 11) was not markedly effective, probably due to the greater tumor burden present at the time of treatment initiation.

TABLE 7 *Response of B16 melanoma to combined cytoxan and OK-432 treatment*

Grp. No.[a]	Cytoxan 200 mg/kg i.p.	OK-432 4 mg/kg i.v.	Liver foci[b] day		Lung foci[c] day		MST[c] (days)	Range of death
			10	20	10	20		
1	—	—	0	60	88	TNTC	21	20–24
2	D-3	—	9	—	96	—	20	19–23
3	—	D-3	0	—	55	—	25	22–27
4	D4	—	—	0	—	65	35	31–45
5	D7	—	—	7	—	140	27	22–35
6	D7	D10	—	0	—	43	32	25 > 60[d]
7	D7, 14	—	—	12	—	54	34	30–41
8	D7, 14	D4, 10	—	0	—	28	39	32 > 60[d]
9	D7, 14	D10, 17	—	0	—	26	41	28 > 60[d]
10	—	D4, 10	—	25	—	52	23	21–28
11	—	D10, 17	—	48	—	185	22	20–25

a) C57BL/6 mice inoculated with 2×10^5 B16 melanoma cells i.v. on day 0.
b) The average number of liver or lung tumor foci counted in mice sacrificed on indicated days.
c) MST = median survival time. All groups contained 20 mice.
d) Ten percent survival on day 60 when experiment was terminated. The results are the average of two separate experiments.

Discussion

The current studies show that OK-432 possesses multifaceted immunomodulatory activity. OK-432 augments NK cell cytotoxicity in vitro and we have confirmed its in vivo activity as previously reported.[11] It activated Mϕ in vitro and in vivo to exert tumoricidal activity against the MBL-2 and P815 tumors, as well as other tumors,[2,12] and as shown in this study and others[13,14] has the capacity to stimulate cytotoxic T lymphocytes. It stimulates the production and secretion of CSF in vivo, as it has also been shown to do in vitro in a clonal SV40-transformed Mϕ line.[15] In addition, it has an influence on inducing hematopoietic spleen colony formation in irradiated mice.[16] OK-432 possesses antitumor therapeutic value when administered alone,[17,18] and also when combined with other cancer treatment modalities.[19,20] One aspect that must be examined in more detail is the depressed NK cell response resulting from multiple treatment as shown in the present study (Table 3). In a clinical study,[11] a significant increase in augmentation of NK cell cytotoxicity was seen in the peripheral blood of cancer patients receiving daily injections, with maximum activity appearing by the third day; however, in spite of successive daily administration, the level of cytotoxicity declined. A similar decrease was also reported in another study in which patients were receiving daily injections.[21]

A considerable number of clinical studies with OK-432 report a therapeutic effect.[3,21-24] A persistent observation has been the excellent NK cell response achieved in peripheral blood, particularly its capacity to augment NK cells in patients with carcinomatous pleural effusions after intrapleural injection.

OK-432 is one of the few agents which has been studied in such detail and found to exert such diverse immunomodulating activity. Results of preclinical and clinical studies indicate that this agent will be of considerable therapeutic value in a combined modality treatment protocol for various human tumors.

References

1. Okamoto, H., Shoin, S. and Koshimura, S. (1978): Streptolysin S-forming and antitumor activities of group A streptococci. In: *Bacterial toxins and cell membranes,* pp. 259. Editors: J. Jeljaszewicz and T. Wadström. Academic Press, London.
2. Ishii, Y., Yamaoka, H., Toh, K. and Kikuchi, K. (1976): Inhibition of tumor growth in vivo and in vitro by macrophages from rats treated with a streptococcal preparation, OK-432. *Gann, 61,* 115.
3. Micksche, M., Kokron, O. and Uchida, A. (1982): Clinical and immunopharmacological studies with OK-432, a streptococcal preparation. In: *Current concepts in human immunology, and cancer immunomodulation,* pp. 639. Editors: B. Serrou, C. Rosenfeld, J.C. Daniels and J.P. Saunders. Elsevier Biomedical Press, B.V., Amsterdam.
4. Herberman, R.B., Nunn, M.E. and Lavrin, D.H. (1975): Natural cytotoxic reac-

tivity of mouse lymphoid cells against syngeneic and allogeneic tumors. I. Distribution of reactivity and specificity. *Int. J. Cancer, 16,* 216.
5. Norbury, K.C. and Fidler, I.J. (1975): In vitro tumor cell destruction by syngeneic mouse macrophages: Methods for assaying cytotoxicity. *J. Immunol. Methods, 7,* 109.
6. Chirigos, M.A., Schlick, E., Piccoli, M., Read, E., Hartung, K. and Bartocci, A. (1983): Characterization of agents. In: *Advances in Immunopharmacology, Vol. II,* pp. 669. Editors: J. Hadden, L. Chedid, P. Dukor, F. Spreafico and D. Willoughby. Pergamon Press, New York.
7. Schlick, E., Bartocci, A. and Chirigos, M.A. (1982): Effect of Azimexone on the bone marrow of normal and γ irradiated mice. *J. Biological Response Modifiers, 1,* 179.
8. Ladisch, S., Reaman, G.H. and Poplack, D.G. (1979): Bacillus Calmette-Guérin enhancement of colony-stimulating activity and myeloid colony formation following administration of cyclophosphamide. *Cancer Res., 39,* 2544.
9. Brunner, K.T., Mauel, J., Cerottini, J. and Chaperis, B. (1968): Quantitative assay of the lytic action of immune lymphoid cells on ^{51}Cr-labelled allogeneic target cells in vitro, inhibition by isoantibody and by drugs. *Immunology, 14,* 181.
10. Henney, C.S. (1971): Quantitation of the cell-mediated immune response. I. The number of cytolytically active mouse lymphoid cells induced by immunization with allogeneic mastocytoma cells. *J. Immunol., 107,* 1558.
11. Oshimi, K., Kano, S., Takaku, F. and Okumura, K. (1980): Augmentation of mouse natural killer cell activity by a streptococcal preparation, OK-432. *J. Natl. Cancer Inst., 65,* 1265.
12. Kawaguchi, T., Suematsu, M., Koizumi, H.M., Mitsui, H., Suzuki, S., Matsuno, T., Ogawa, H. and Nomoto, K. (1983): Activation of macrophage function by intraperitoneal administration of the streptococcal antitumor agent OK-432. *Immunopharmacology, 6,* 1977.
13. Kai, S., Tanaka, J., Nomoto, K. and Torisu, M. (1979): Studies on the immunopotentiating effects of a streptococcal preparation, OK-432. *Clin. Exp. Immunol., 37,* 98.
14. Hojo, H. and Hashimoto, Y. (1981): Cytotoxic cells induced in tumor-bearing rats by a streptococcal preparation (OK-432). *Gann, 72,* 692.
15. Takayama, H., Tanigawa, T. and Takagi, A. (1981): Production of interferon by an SV40-transformed macrophage line, BB-W-531-2. *Microbiol. Immunol., 25,* 683.
16. Hiraoka, A., Yamagishi, M., Ohkubo, T., Kamamoto, T., Yoshida, Y. and Uchino, H. (1981): Effect of a streptococcal preparation, OK-432, on hematopoietic spleen colony formation in irradiated mice. *Cancer Res., 41,* 2954.
17. Aoki, T., Kvedar, J.P., Hollis, Jr. V.W. and Bushar, G.S. (1976): Brief communicaion: Streptococcus pyogenes preparation OK-432: Immunoprophylactic and immunotherapeutic effects on the incidence of spontaneous leukemia in AKR mice. *J. Natl. Cancer Inst., 56,* 687.
18. Sakurai, Y., Tsukagoshi, S., Satoh, H., Akiba, T., Suzuki, S. and Takagaki, Y. (1972): Tumor-inhibitory effect of a streptococcal preparation (NSC-B116209). *Cancer Chemother. Rep., 56,* 9.
19. Yamagata, S., Koh, T., Oride, M. and Hattori, T. (1980): Antitumor effects of levamisole in combination with anaerobic corynebacterium, OK-432 (streptococcal preparation), and chemotherapy in mice. *Cancer Immunol. Immunother., 7,* 217.
20. Mashiba, H., Matsunaga, K. and Gojobori, M. (1979): Effect of immunochemotherapy with OK-432 and yeast cell wall on the activities of peritoneal

macrophages of mice. *Gann, 70,* 687.
21. Wakasugi, H., Oshimi, K., Miyata, M. and Morioka, Y. (1981): Augmentation of natural killer (NK) cell activity by a streptococcal preparation, OK-432, in patients with malignant tumors. *Clin. Immunol., 1,* 154.
22. Uchida, A. and Micksche, M. (1983): Intrapleural administration of OK-432 in cancer patients: Activation of NK cells and reduction of suppressor cells.
23. Uchida, A. and Hoshino, T. (1980a): Clinical studies on cell-mediated immunity in patients with malignant disease. *Cancer, 45,* 476.
24. Uchida, A. and Hoshino, T. (1980b): Reduction of suppressor cells in cancer patients treated with OK-432 immunotherapy. *Int. J. Cancer, 26,* 401.

The effects of OK-432 on porcine NK and K cell system

YOON BERM KIM*

Sloan-Kettering Institute for Cancer Research, Memorial Sloan-Kettering Cancer Center, Rye, NY, U.S.A.

Introduction

In light of the potential importance of the natural killer (NK) and killer (K) cell system in the host defense mechanisms against neoplastic growth and tumor metastasis as well as viral infections, we have been investigating the ontogenic development, cellular nature and lineages, and regulatory mechanisms for NK activity in our gnotobiotic miniature swine by taking advantage of the fact that immunologically ''virgin'' piglets would not be contaminated with ''natural'' antibodies in vivo, and that they could be maintained in a controlled environment.[1] We have found that K cells for antibody-dependent cellular cytotoxicity (ADCC) develop early in ontogeny, and before the development of NK cells, that NK and K cells have different tissue distributions, that NK cells are not K cells armed with ''natural'' antibodies, and that heterologous ''anti-NK'' sera plus C' eliminate NK cells without affecting ADCC, suggesting that porcine NK cells and K cells are distinct subpopulations.[2,3-5] This is further supported by the differential effects of interferons on NK and ADCC, and the differential effects of recently developed monoclonal antibodies against NK cells on NK and K cells.[6,7]

We found that NK cells develop two weeks and three to four weeks after birth in specific pathogen-free (SPF) and germfree (GF) piglets respectively. When GF piglets were associated with anaerobic flora (Lactobacillus sp. and Streptococcus sp. from SPF swine), they developed significant NK activity within two weeks of age, indicating that microbial flora is responsible for acceleration of maturation or differentiation of NK cells during ontogeny.[5,8] Since OK-432, a streptococcal preparation (Picibanil, Chugai Pharmaceutical Co., Ltd., Tokyo, Japan), has been reported to be a potent augmentor of human NK cell activity because it activates NK cells and reduces suppressor cells,[9-11] we have examined the effects of OK-432 on our porcine

*Present address: Department of Microbiology and Immunology, University of Health Sciences, The Chicago Medical School, North Chicago, IL, U.S.A.

NK and K cell system in vitro as well as in vivo to investigate the regulation of NK and K cell activities.

Materials and methods

Animals: GF, colostrum-deprived piglets, obtained by aseptic hysterectomy three to five days prior to term from SPF miniature sows, were maintained in GF isolators on a diet of sterile water and soybean milk. Naturally-farrowed, colostrum-fed, SPF piglets were maintained in our SPF facility with HEPA filter filtered air, chlorinated water and autoclaved feed were used for these experiments.

Preparation of lymphoid cells, culture systems and removal of adherent cells: These are described in detail elsewhere.[3]

Target cell preparation: Human erythroid leukemia cell line K562 for NK targets and human B-cell line SB modified with 2,4,6-trinitrobenzene sulfonate (TNP-SB) and porcine anti-TNP sera for ADCC targets were used for the NK and ADCC assay as described elsewhere.[3]

Assay for NK and ADCC and calculation of cytotoxic activity: A four-hour ^{51}Cr-release assay method was used to determine cytotoxic activities for both NK and ADCC as described elsewhere.[3] All assays were done with effector-to-target ratios of 100:1, 50:1 and 25:1. For the sake of simplicity, these are not shown in all tables.

OK-432: OK-432 was kindly supplied by Chugai Pharmaceutical Co., Ltd., Tokyo, Japan. Vials containing 5 KE (0.5 mg dried streptococci) OK-432 were pooled and washed in sterile saline two times and resuspended in a sterile balanced salt solution (BSS) at the concentration of 1.0 mg/ml. This stock solution was used for these experiments.

Results

Establishment of the optimal effective dose and time of incubation to study the effects of OK-432 on porcine NK and K cell activities in vitro

Table 1 shows that an in vitro preincubation of OK-432 with PBL from young adult SPF miniature swine gave a dose-dependent augmentation of NK activity. The maximum augmentation was observed with 50 μg/ml in culture. However, there was little effect on ADCC at any dose level. Kinetic studies on augmentation of NK activity by OK-432 treated effector cells which were given the predetermined optimum dose of 50 μg/ml showed that an 18-hour, 37°C culture gave a maximum response (Table 2). Once again there was little effect on ADCC. Addition of OK-432 directly in the assay mixture had little effect on NK and ADCC. Monocytes were not required for augmentation of NK activity by OK-432. This was demonstrated by the equal enhancement of NK activity of unseparated peripheral blood mononuclear cells (PBM), and of monocyte-depleted PBL, both of which were incubated with OK-432 for 18 hours at 37°C (Table 3).

Effect of OK-432 on porcine NK and K cell activities in vitro

Table 4 shows that OK-432 augmented NK activity at least two fold in PBL of all 12 SPF miniature swine. In contrast, only four of the 12 tested (SPF 4117-6, SPF 4135-5, SPF 4147-3 and SPF 4155-6) had some augmentation of ADCC; the rest had no significant change or slightly depressed ADCC. These results indicate that OK-432 specifically augments NK cell activity but not K cell activity.

TABLE 1 *Titration of effects of OK-432 on porcine NK and K cell activities in vitro*

Animal no.	OK-432[a) (μg/ml)	% Specific lysis[b)		
		K562	TNP-SB	TNP-SB + anti-TNP
SPF 4127–2	0 (Control)	24.5 ± 2.1	6.5 ± 0.2	41.4 ± 2.7
	0.05	23.1 ± 1.3	5.3 ± 0.2	41.4 ± 1.1
	0.5	30.8 ± 0.6	7.7 ± 0.4	41.7 ± 0.9
	5.0	34.4 ± 1.7	12.7 ± 2.2	41.7 ± 1.1
	50.0	42.1 ± 3.0	7.8 ± 2.1	45.3 ± 1.2
SPF 4135–6	0 (Control)	21.0 ± 0.8	4.2 ± 0.3	72.5 ± 0.3
	0.05	33.5 ± 0.7	4.5 ± 0.6	72.2 ± 0.9
	0.5	37.2 ± 1.5	4.7 ± 0.3	54.6 ± 3.6
	5.0	47.9 ± 1.1	4.5 ± 1.0	66.2 ± 2.4
	50.0	46.7 ± 2.8	5.1 ± 0.7	63.4 ± 2.1
SPF 4166–3	0 (Control)	36.3 ± 2.9	3.5 ± 0.4	86.5 ± 4.4
	0.05	46.9 ± 4.6	2.9 ± 0.6	96.3 ± 2.7
	0.5	50.9 ± 2.9	3.8 ± 0.1	90.5 ± 2.3
	5.0	56.5 ± 1.7	3.4 ± 1.6	94.0 ± 3.6
	50.0	63.3 ± 2.1	2.8 ± 1.7	93.1 ± 3.3
SPF 4135–1	0 (Control)	12.6 ± 0.5	2.1 ± 2.4	53.7 ± 4.2
	0.05	18.8 ± 2.4	2.2 ± 1.3	63.9 ± 1.4
	0.5	21.7 ± 0.8	3.1 ± 1.8	53.1 ± 2.2
	5.0	24.1 ± 1.5	2.2 ± 1.1	56.0 ± 2.7
	50.0	30.8 ± 1.0	3.9 ± 3.0	60.6 ± 2.8

a) PBL from SPF miniature swine were incubated with varying concentrations of OK-432 for 18 hr at 37°C and washed three times with BSS before assay.
b) Effector-to-target ratios were 100:1.

TABLE 2 *Pretreatment of effector cells with OK-432 for varying time period for its effects on NK and K cell activities*

Animal no.	Treatment of effectors[a]	% Specific lysis[b]		
		K562	TNP-SB	TNP-SB + anti-TNP
SPF 4119–5	PBL Control	31.1 ± 2.9	7.7 ± 2.3	58.9 ± 1.0
	PBL + OK-432 0 hr, washed	36.7 ± 4.2	9.2 ± 0.7	54.3 ± 2.3
	PBL + OK-432 3 hr, washed	40.9 ± 2.7	7.8 ± 2.2	58.3 ± 3.8
	PBL + OK-432 18 hr, washed	63.9 ± 11.0	19.3 ± 0.8	66.7 ± 0.9
	PBL + OK-432 in assay	30.8 ± 2.2	4.4 ± 0.2	59.9 ± 1.7
SPF 4135–5	PBL Control	6.6 ± 2.8	0.9 ± 0.3	28.9 ± 1.7
	PBL + OK-432 0 hr, washed	8.8 ± 2.0	0.8 ± 0.0	35.3 ± 5.8
	PBL + OK-432 3 hr, washed	9.4 ± 1.3	1.6 ± 0.1	31.0 ± 0.5
	PBL + OK-432 18 hr, washed	27.4 ± 3.0	2.4 ± 0.7	49.8 ± 0.7
	PBL + OK-432 in assay	13.1 ± 0.0	0.4 ± 0.3	37.4 ± 1.3
SPF 4177–2	PBL Control	17.7 ± 2.8	2.2 ± 0.4	61.2 ± 2.9
	PBL + OK-432 0 hr, washed	17.1 ± 0.2	1.8 ± 0.2	54.2 ± 5.8
	PBL + OK-432 3 hr, washed	18.1 ± 0.5	2.2 ± 0.9	59.4 ± 2.1
	PBL + OK-432 18 hr, washed	43.5 ± 3.4	2.7 ± 1.0	55.7 ± 3.1
	PBL + OK-432 in assay	19.2 ± 2.0	0.4 ± 0.6	50.9 ± 1.9

a) PBL from SPF miniature swine were incubated with medium (control) or OK-432 50 μg/ml for 0, 3 or 18 hr at 37°C and washed three times with BSS before assay or OK-432 50 μg/ml was added directly into assay mixture.
b) Effector-to-target ratios were 100:1.

TABLE 3 *Role of monocytes on NK augmenting effects of OK-432 on porcine PBL*

Animal no.	Treatment of effectors[a]	% Specific lysis[b]		
		K562	TNP-SB	TNP-SB + anti-TNP
SPF 4135–1	PBM Control	27.4 ± 2.3	7.5 ± 1.9	55.2 ± 0.9
	PBM + OK-432	50.8 ± 2.0	13.4 ± 0.5	68.9 ± 2.8
	PBL Control	18.5 ± 1.9	5.3 ± 1.2	44.8 ± 1.7
	PBL + OK-432	54.6 ± 1.2	19.1 ± 4.5	74.8 ± 1.4
SPF 4172–3	PBM Control	32.9 ± 1.5	23.8 ± 1.1	72.1 ± 3.3
	PBM + OK-432	48.9 ± 1.5	25.5 ± 2.4	64.2 ± 2.8
	PBL Control	38.2 ± 2.6	2.2 ± 0.8	86.6 ± 0.7
	PBL + OK-432	43.3 ± 2.7	22.5 ± 1.3	70.3 ± 2.2

a) Peripheral blood mononuclear cells not depleted of monocytes (PBM) or depleted of monocytes by removal of adherent cells (PBL) were incubated with medium (control) or OK-432 50 μg-ml for 18 hr at 37°C and washed three times with BSS before assay.
b) Effector-to-target ratios were 100:1.

TABLE 4 *Effect of OK-432 on porcine NK and K cell activities in vitro*

Animal no.	% Specific lysis[a)			
	NK (K562)		ADCC (TNP-SB + anti-TNP)	
	Control	OK-432	Control	OK-432
SPF 4108–7	7.8 ± 1.0	14.5 ± 2.5	73.2 ± 1.6	64.3 ± 2.2
SPF 4117–3	12.6 ± 0.6	23.0 ± 2.7	57.2 ± 5.1	52.2 ± 2.7
SPF 4117–6	14.8 ± 2.1	32.9 ± 0.8	60.8 ± 4.7	72.5 ± 4.7
SPF 4119–5	31.1 ± 2.9	63.8 ± 4.1	58.9 ± 1.0	66.7 ± 0.8
SPF 4127–2	24.5 ± 2.1	42.1 ± 3.0	41.4 ± 2.7	45.3 ± 1.2
SPF 4135–1	12.6 ± 0.5	30.8 ± 1.0	53.7 ± 4.2	60.6 ± 2.8
SPF 4135–5	15.5 ± 5.5	39.2 ± 8.5	46.2 ± 3.8	62.7 ± 3.1
SPF 4135–6	21.1 ± 0.8	46.7 ± 2.8	72.5 ± 0.3	63.4 ± 2.1
SPF 4147–3	12.0 ± 0.5	46.5 ± 3.5	49.3 ± 2.5	77.1 ± 10.4
SPF 4155–6	9.1 ± 1.4	19.9 ± 1.6	24.4 ± 0.8	36.0 ± 0.3
SPF 4166–3	17.2 ± 2.9	45.9 ± 4.0	81.5 ± 2.9	78.1 ± 2.9
SPF 4172–2	23.1 ± 1.8	64.2 ± 3.2	78.0 ± 3.1	71.2 ± 1.1

a) PBL from SPF miniature swine were incubated with medium (control) or OK-432 50 μg/ml for 18 hr at 37°C and washed three times with BSS before assay. Effector-to-target ratios were 100:1.

TABLE 5 *Induction of NK activity of PBL from neonatal piglet by OK-432 in vitro*

Treatment of effectors[a)	E:T ratios	% Specific lysis		
		K562	TNP-SB	TNP-SB + anti-TNP
PBL control	100:1	2.6 ± 1.0	1.9 ± 0.5	77.5 ± 5.0
	50:1	1.7 ± 0.2	−0.5 ± 0.6	70.4 ± 6.4
	25:1	1.4 ± 1.1	−0.3 ± 0.3	66.2 ± 1.5
PBL + OK-432	100:1	43.5 ± 0.9	2.0 ± 0.2	75.8 ± 2.2
(50 μg/ml)	50:1	25.5 ± 0.6	0.9 ± 0.2	71.7 ± 3.1
	25:1	13.3 ± 1.5	−0.6 ± 0.8	55.6 ± 2.1
Spleen control	100:1	−0.3 ± 0.6	0.1 ± 1.3	98.2 ± 3.3
	50:1	−0.6 ± 0.4	−0.3 ± 0.5	101.5 ± 3.6
	25:1	1.9 ± 1.3	−0.4 ± 0.4	87.1 ± 5.0
Spleen + OK-432	100:1	0.8 ± 1.1	−0.9 ± 0.2	78.3 ± 1.8
(50 μg/ml)	50:1	0.9 ± 1.7	−0.4 ± 0.7	75.3 ± 3.0
	25:1	−0.2 ± 0.4	−0.7 ± 0.5	84.7 ± 10.6

a) PBL or spleen cells of 0-day-old piglet (SPF 4178–1) were incubated with medium (control) or OK-432 50 μg/ml for 3 days at 37°C and washed three times with BSS before assay.

Induction of NK activity of PBL from neonatal piglets by OK-432 in vitro

Table 5 shows that when PBL of "background-free" neonatal piglets were incubated with OK-432 for three days in vitro NK activity was induced. The same incubation of spleen cells from the same animals however did not induce NK activity. These data indicate that OK-432 is a potent inducer of NK cells, and that inducible pre-NK cells are present in neonatal blood but not in their spleens.

In vivo effects of OK-432 on NK activity of gnotobiotic and GF immunologically "virgin" piglets

When "background-positive" gnotobiotic piglets were injected intraperitoneally with 1.0 mg of OK-432, there was a significant augmentation of NK activity within 3 days post-injection. This activity returned to pre-injection levels at day 6 (Table 6). When background-free GF, immunologically "virgin" piglets were injected intraperitoneally with 0.5 to 1.0 mg of OK-432, there was a significant acceleration in the induction of NK activity within three to 13 days post-injection (Table 7). Although the number of animals was small, it appears that intraperitoneal injection is superior to intradermal injection of OK-432 for induction of NK activity.

Discussion

The streptococcal preparation OK-432 (Picibanil, Chugai Pharmaceutical Co., Ltd., Tokyo, Japan) is prepared by incubating the culture of low-virulent Su strain of *Streptococcus pyogenes* of human origin, treated with penicillin G potassium. This incubation mixture is then heated at 45°C for 30 minutes, and subsequently lyophilized. OK-432 is a potent biological response modifier,[12] which augments human NK activity by both activation of NK cells and reduction of suppressor cells.[9-11] OK-432 has been used as an immunotherapeutic drug either alone or in combination with chemotherapy and radiotherapy of various cancer patients with impressive success in Japan.[12]

Since we were interested in investigating the ontogeny and regulation of NK and K cell systems in our gnotobiotic miniature swine system, we searched for various biological response modifier drugs for our studies. OK-432 was reported to be a potent augmentor of human NK activity by both activation of NK cells and reduction of suppressor cells by Uchida et al.[9-11] This prompted us to examine the effects of OK-432 on our porcine NK and K cell system. It has been observed that preincubation of effectors for 18 hours at 37°C with 5 to 50 μg/ml of OK-432 is required for the optimal augmentation of NK activity from the PBL from SPF swine who

TABLE 6 *In vivo effects of OK-432 on NK cell activity of gnotobiotic piglets*

Animal no.	Treatment[a)]	E:T ratios	% Specific lysis (K562)[b)]			
			Day 0	Day 3	Day 6	Day 13
XGF 4165–1	Control	100:1	32.6 ± 3.4	33.0 ± 5.4	21.6 ± 0.6	26.9 ± 1.5
		50:1	27.3 ± 4.8	23.7 ± 2.6	8.0 ± 0.2	13.8 ± 0.6
		25:1	12.3 ± 1.3	12.4 ± 1.8	2.4 ± 0.6	5.0 ± 1.6
XGF 4165–5	Control	100:1	6.3 ± 2.2	15.2 ± 0.0	15.3 ± 0.8	12.9 ± 1.3
		50:1	5.7 ± 0.6	9.2 ± 0.0	7.9 ± 1.1	8.0 ± 1.8
		25:1	2.8 ± 0.2	9.0 ± 0.0	1.8 ± 0.3	0.9 ± 0.8
XGF 4165–2	OK-432	100:1	19.8 ± 0.9	61.7 ± 2.1	24.9 ± 0.2	26.7 ± 3.2
		50:1	8.2 ± 0.1	38.9 ± 0.8	10.8 ± 0.7	12.0 ± 1.2
		25:1	4.0 ± 0.1	14.0 ± 1.8	3.8 ± 0.6	4.9 ± 0.7
XGF 4165–8	OK-432	100:1	37.6 ± 2.3	61.7 ± 3.4	40.4 ± 1.8	22.7 ± 2.3
		50:1	22.6 ± 1.3	44.9 ± 3.8	20.5 ± 1.3	8.5 ± 0.9
		25:1	12.1 ± 0.7	22.4 ± 1.5	7.6 ± 0.5	1.7 ± 0.5

a) Four littermates of 5-month-old gnotobiotic (mono-contaminated) piglets were divided into two groups: one injected with OK-432 1.0 mg intraperitoneally and others were uninjected (controls).
b) NK assay on PBL from piglets of preinjection (Day 0), and Days 3, 6 and 13 after the injection.

TABLE 7 *In vivo effects of OK-432 on ontogeny of NK cells of germfree immunologically "virgin" piglets*

Animal no.	Treatment[a)]	% Specific lysis (K562)[b)] Day 3		Day 13	
		100:1	50:1	100:1	50:1
GF 4182–7	Control	0.7 ± 1.2	−0.9 ± 0.3	2.4 ± 1.1	1.1 ± 1.1
GF 4182–1	OK-432 (1 mg, i.p.)	5.5 ± 0.4	2.6 ± 0.9	4.9 ± 0.7	2.2 ± 0.3
GF 4182–2	OK-432 (1 mg, i.p.)	12.8 ± 3.1	8.8 ± 1.4	41.7 ± 4.0	25.7 ± 3.1
GF 4182–4	OK-432 (1 mg, i.d.)	2.6 ± 1.5	0.8 ± 1.3	5.2 ± 1.4	1.3 ± 0.5
GF 4182–6	OK-432 (1 mg, i.d.)	0.5 ± 0.5	0.6 ± 1.3	6.8 ± 0.8	2.3 ± 1.2
GF 4187–6	Control	1.1 ± 2.1	0.0 ± 0.3		
GF 4187–7	Control	2.9 ± 1.7	2.8 ± 0.6		
GF 4187–1	OK-432 (0.5 mg, i.p.)	7.4 ± 0.8	5.5 ± 0.6		
GF 4187–2	OK-432 (0.5 mg, i.p.)	7.5 ± 2.4	4.1 ± 2.1		

a) Germfree colostrum deprived, immunologically "virgin" piglets (0 day of age) were injected with OK-432, 1.0 mg intraperitoneally (i.p.) or intradermally (i.d.) or 0.5 mg i.p., or uninjected (controls).
b) NK assay on PBL from GF piglets of days 3 and 13 after the injection.

have pre-existing NK cells and three days of incubation is required for induction of NK activity from background-free newborn piglets (Tables 1, 2, 4 and 5). This is unlike interferon which requires very short-term incubation (three hours) for the maximum effects. The fact that OK-432 requires 18 hours or longer of incubation time for the maximum augmentation of NK activity to occur, indicates that OK-432 may not work directly on NK cells, but it may be a mediator for induction of interferons, interleukins and/or NK activating factors.[13] These, in turn, may stimulate NK cells or induce pre-NK cells to become active NK cells. This is supported further by the results obtained in in vivo effects of OK-432 on NK activity of gnotobiotic and GF piglets, since it took days to get the maximum augmentation and/or induction of NK activity (Tables 6 and 7).

Our results on the effects of OK-432 on porcine NK and K cell systems agree with the findings of many studies on human NK cells.[9-11,14] This suggests that swine, which are physiologically very similar to humans, may provide an ideal animal model with which to investigate further the effects of OK-432 on the host defense system. Although the exact mechanisms of activation and/or induction of differentiation of NK cells by OK-432 are not known, it is clear that OK-432 does more than simply induce interferons. This was indicated by the fact that the purified interferons augmented only pre-existing NK cell activity but failed to induce NK activity of PBL from less than 3-week-old GF piglets whose NK activity had not yet developed.[6,15] In contrast, OK-432 induced NK activity in vitro as well as in vivo from background-free newborn piglets (Tables 5 and 7). Perhaps OK-432 acts very similarly to living microbial associations in GF piglets.[5,8] The NK activating factor induction by OK-432 may be one of the mechanisms which induced NK activity from background-free newborn piglets.[13] These results support that OK-432 is indeed a good biological response modifier, particularly in regulation of porcine NK cell activity.

Summary and conclusion

The streptococcal preparation OK-432 (Picibanil, Chugai Pharmaceutical Co., Ltd., Tokyo, Japan) augmented porcine NK activity in vitro as well as in vivo, but had little effect on ADCC. OK-432 is also a strong inducer of neonatal NK cells. Thus, OK-432 is a good biological response modifier, particularly in regulation of porcine NK cell activity.

Acknowledgments

The author wishes to acknowledge the assistance of Mr. Donald C. Moody for procuring animals for this study; Mr. Gene A. Monson for his excellent technical assistance, and Mrs. Rose Vecchiolla for the preparation of the manuscript.

References

1. Kim, Y.B. (1975): Developmental immunity in the piglet. In: *Immunodeficiency Diseases in Man and Animals.* The National Foundation-March of Dimes, Birth Defects Original Article Series, Vol. XI, No. 1, pp. 549. Editors: D. Bergsma, R.A. Good and J. Finstad. Sinauer Associates, Inc., Sunderland, Massachusetts.
2. Huh, N.D. Kim, Y.B. and Amos, D.B.(1981): Natural killing (NK) and antibody-dependent cellular cytotoxicity (ADCC) in specific pathogen-free (SPF) miniature swine and germfree piglets. III. Two distinct effector cells for NK and ADCC. *J. Immunol., 127,* 2190.
3. Kim, Y.B., Huh, N.D., Koren, H.S. and Amos, D.B. (1980): Natural killing (NK) and antibody-dependent cellular cytotoxicity (ADCC) in specific pathogen-free (SPF) miniature swine and germfree piglets. I. Comparison of NK and ADCC. *J. Immunol., 125,* 755.
4. Kim, Y.B. and Huh, N.D. (1981): Natural killer and killer (NK/K) cell system in gnotobiotic miniature swine. In: *Recent Advances in Germfree Research,* pp. 585. Editors: S. Sasaki, A. Ozawa and K. Hashimoto. Tokai University Press, Tokyo.
5. Kim, Y.B., Huh, N.D., Koren, H.S. and Amos, D.B. (1982): Ontogenic development of porcine NK and K cells. In: *NK Cells and Other Natural Effector Cells,* pp. 341. Editor: R.B. Herberman. Academic Press, New York.
6. Chung, T.J., Huh, N.D. and Kim, Y.B. (1982): Differential effects of interferons on porcine NK and K cell activities. In: *NK Cells and Other Natural Effector Cells,* pp. 381. Editor: R.B. Herberman. Academic Press, New York.
7. Kim, Y.B., Czajkowski, M. and Monson, G.A. (1984): Distinct subpopulations of NK and K cells in porcine natural cell-mediated immunity. In: *Natural Killer Activity and Its Regulation,* pp. 250. Editors: T. Hoshino, H.S. Koren and A. Uchida. Excerpta Medica, Tokyo.
8. Huh, N.D., Kim, Y.B., Koren, H.S. and Amos, D.B. (1981): Natural killing and antibody-dependent cellular cytotoxicity in specific pathogen-free miniature swine and germfree piglets. II. Ontogenic development of NK and ADCC. *Int. J. Cancer, 23,* 175.
9. Uchida, A. and Hoshino, T. (1980): Reduction of suppressor cells in cancer patients treated with OK-432 immunotherapy. *Int. J. Cancer, 26,* 401.
10. Uchida, A. and Micksche, M. (1981): In vitro augmentation of natural killing activity by OK-432. *Int. J. Immunopharm., 3,* 365.
11. Uchida, A. and Micksche, M. (1983): Intrapleural administration of OK-432 in cancer patients: Activation of NK cells and reduction of suppressor cells. *Int. J. Cancer, 31,* 1.
12. Ishida, N., Hoshino, T. and Uchida, A. (1983): A Streptococcal Preparation as a Potent Biological Response Modifier-OK-432. Excerpta Medica, Amsterdam-Princeton-Geneva-Tokyo.
13. Ichimura, O., Suzuki, S., Sugawara, Y., Fukui, H., Shitara, K. and Osawa, T. (1983): Characterization of mouse natural killer cell activating factor (NKAF) induced by streptococcal preparation OK-432: Evidence for interferon and interleukin 2 independent NK cell activation. *Br. J. Cancer.* (Submitted for publication).
14. Moore, M., Kimber, I. and Bakacs, T. (1984): Differential activity of OK-432 on natural killer (NK) activity and antibody-dependent cellular cytotoxicity (ADCC). In: *Proceedings of International Symposium on OK-432,* pp. 40. Editors: T. Hoshino and A. Uchida. Excerpta Medica, Tokyo.

15. Chung, T.J. and Kim, Y.B. (1983): Effect of recombinant human leukocyte interferons on porcine NK and K cell activities. *In: Interferons as Modulators of Immune System*. Workshop No. 403-12, 5th International Congress of Immunology, Kyoto, Japan.

Differential activity of OK-432 on natural killer (NK) activity and antibody-dependent cellular cytotoxicity (ADCC)

MICHAEL MOORE[1], IAN KIMBER[2] and TIBOR BAKACS[3]

[1]*Department of Immunology, Paterson Laboratories, Christie Hospital and Holt Radium Institute, Manchester,* [2]*Immunology Section, ICI Central Toxicology Laboratory, Cheshire, U.K. and* [3]*National Institute of Oncology, Budapest, Hungary*

Introduction

A distinction exists between human peripheral blood and other secondary lymphoid organs with respect to levels of basal natural killer/killer (NK/K) cell activities and responses to various immunomodulators including some of current clinical interest.[1-3] Such differences are exemplified by the apparent failure of IFN-α to induce or enhance NK activity in tonsillar lymphocytes,[1] or to influence K cell lysis or sensitized human erythrocytes,[4] reflecting heterogeneity among NK/K cells either with respect to cell type and lineage or to functional/maturational status. Other immunomodulators, however, including Staphylococcal enterotoxin A (SEA), a potent mitogen and inducer of IFN-γ,[5] and supernatants derived from polyclonally-activated human lymphocytes, possess the capability to enhance both NK and K cell functions under conditions where IFN-α is ineffective.[1,6] In an attempt to further elucidate the factors which regulate NK and K cell functions, we have recently begun to examine the efficacy of an anti-tumor pharmaceutical preparation of a low virulent Su strain of *Streptococcus pyogenes* (OK-432) which purportedly induces IFN (α and γ) and interleukin-2 (IL-2).[7] The data may have implications for the subtypes of killer cells which are responsive to different immunomodulators and the mechanisms by which these cells are activated.

Materials and methods

Immunomodulators: OK-432 was supplied by the Chugai Pharmaceutical Co., Ltd., Tokyo, Japan, as lyophilized organisms; 1 KE (Klinische Einheit) unit corresponding to 0.1 mg dried streptococci. SEA and gene-cloned IFN-α

2 (Sp-Act 1.6 x 10^8 IU mg^{-1}) were gifts from Dr. A.G. Morris (Warwick University, U.K.) and Dr. C. Weissman (Universität Zurich, Switzerland) respectively.

Effector cells: Peripheral blood lymphocytes (PBL) were obtained from normal volunteers. Lymph node cells (LNC) were obtained from the mesentery of patients undergoing laparotomy for non-neoplastic disease, and tonsillar lymphocytes were taken from juveniles undergoing tonsillectomy for recurrent infection. Procedures for collection, isolation and pretreatment with immunomodulators have been previously described in detail.[1,4,8]

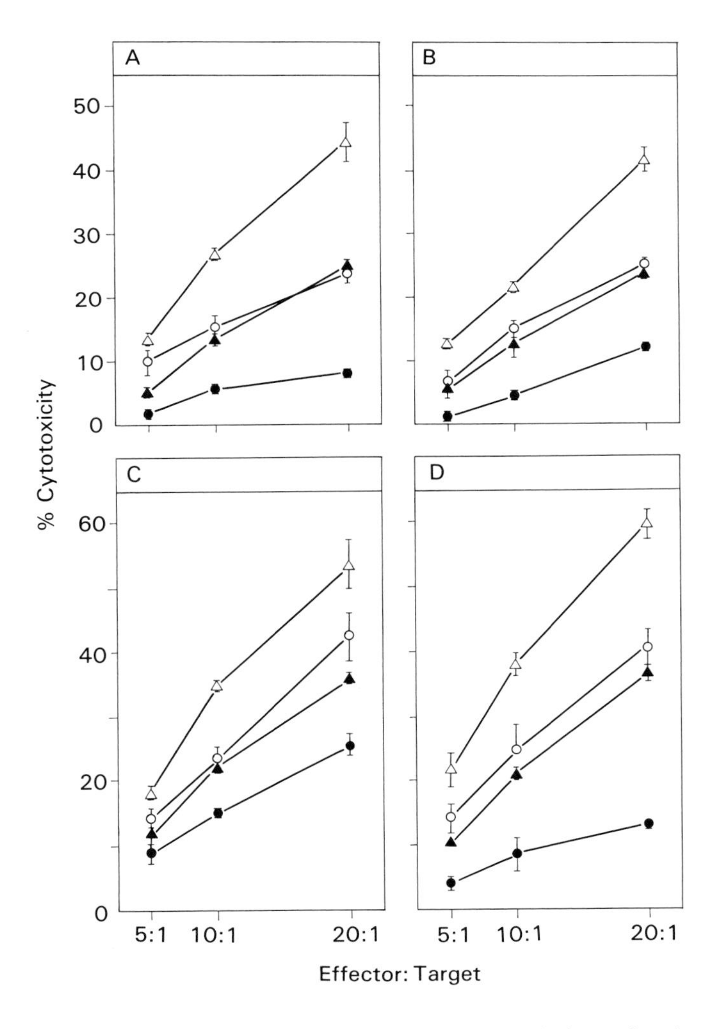

FIGURE 1 *Cytotoxicity against sensitive (E10; open symbols) and resistant (F9; closed symbols) clones of K562 cells by OK-432 treated (triangles) and untreated (circles) PBL.*

Cytotoxicity: NK and K cell activities were determined by lysis of radiolabelled erythroleukemic K562 cells and antibody-coated human red cells respectively. In the latter assay papain-treated O Rh (D) +ve erythrocytes were sensitized with the IgG fraction of pooled anti-D sera.[6] This assay measures ADCC exclusively since unsensitized human erythrocytes under the conditions of these tests are totally resistant to NK.[4] Assays were routinely terminated after 18 hours and data are presented as percentage cytotoxicity, calculated as previously described.[8]

Results

Effect of OK-432 on PBL-NK: Preparatory to investigating the immunoenhancing potential of OK-432 on extravascular NK function and peripheral blood K cell activity, the conditions under which the agent enhanced the activity of PBL-NK were optimized against sensitive (E10) and resistant (F9) clones of the K562 cell line.[9] For this purpose effectors (2×10^6 ml^{-1}) were pretreated for 1 to 18 hours with OK-432 concentrations from 0.01 to 2.5 $KEml^{-1}$. Maximal lysis was achieved following 18 hours of pretreatment with 0.2 KE OK-432 ml-1. Cytotoxicity data obtained under these conditions for four independent donors (A - D) are shown in Figure 1. These levels of activation were comparable with those previously reported for IFN-α and IFN-α2 on PBL-NK.[2,8]

TABLE 1 *Lysis of K562 by tonsillar lymphocytes: Influence of pretreatment with OK-432 and IFN-α2*

		% Cytotoxicity ± S.D.		
Donor	E:T[a)]	RPMI-CS[b)]	IFN-α2[c)]	OK-432[d)]
1	100:1	15.9 ± 2.0	16.4 ± 3.3	29.2 ± 2.0
	50:1	10.0 ± 3.7	7.0 ± 1.6	16.6 ± 0.7
	25:1	4.1 ± 0.3	4.1 ± 2.2	11.5 ± 2.7
2	100:1	14.2 ± 1.2	15.6 ± 3.0	28.0 ± 1.6
	50:1	7.9 ± 1.7	8.4 ± 1.1	18.6 ± 1.4
	25:1	4.0 ± 1.8	6.4 ± 0.7	11.7 ± 3.1
3	100:1	19.4 ± 1.7	17.1 ± 1.0	35.2 ± 1.3
	50:1	12.3 ± 1.3	10.1 ± 1.7	25.1 ± 2.0
	25:1	7.4 ± 0.8	4.9 ± 2.0	14.2 ± 1.2

a) Effector:target ratios. Effector cells treated for 18 hours with b) RPMI-CS, c) 500 $u.ml^{-1}$ IFN-α2 or d) 0.2 $u.ml^{-1}$ OK-432.

Effect of OK-432 on tonsillar NK: The low basal level of NK activity (measured against the parental K562 cell line) necessitated the use of higher E:T ratios (in the range 25:1 to 100:1) than for PBL. In concordance with previous studies, IFN-α2 failed to increase anti-K562 activity (Table 1). OK-432, however, induced levels of cytotoxicity which approached those generated in tonsillar lymphocytes by pretreatment with SEA or supernatants from polyclonally-activated allogenic tonsils.

Effect of OK-432 on LNC-NK: By contrast with tonsillar lymphocytes, basal levels of anti-K562 activity were more variable, as typified by the values for the two patients in Table 2. Although IFN-α2 was again without in-

TABLE 2 *Lysis of K562 by LNC: Influence of pretreatment with IFN-α2, OK-432 and SEA*

		% Cytotoxicity ± S.D.			
Donor	E:T[a]	RPMI-CS[b]	IFN-α2[c]	OK-432[d]	SEA[e]
1	40:1	9.5 ± 1.1	8.2 ± 1.3	18.8 ± 2.0	26.4 ± 0.7
2	80:1	48.9 ± 2.0	47.2 ± 1.7	70.9 ± 2.3	76.2 ± 3.0

a) Effector: target ratio. Effector cells treated for 18 hours with b) RPMI-CS, c) 500 u.ml^{-1} IFN-α2, d) 0.2 u.ml^{-1} OK-432 or e) 0.1 μg ml^{-1} SEA.

TABLE 3 *Natural and antibody-dependent cellular cytotoxicity mediated by peripheral blood lymphocytes: Influence of OK-432*

Donor		% Cytotoxicity ± S.D.			
		NK[c]	ADCC[d] 1/800	ADCC[d] 1/1600	ADCC[d] 1/3200
1	RPMI-CS[a]	40.3 ± 2.9	7.2 ± 0.1	4.8 ± 0.2	2.1 ± 0.1
	OK-432[b]	59.3 ± 2.2	8.7 ± 0.1	6.7 ± 0.4	3.5 ± 0.3
2	RPMI-CS	24.8 ± 1.3	17.4 ± 0.7	13.1 ± 0.1	8.5 ± 0.2
	OK-432	41.7 ± 1.7	12.7 ± 0.1	10.9 ± 0.6	8.4 ± 1.0
3	RPMI-CS	23.7 ± 1.2	42.8 ± 0.7	45.3 ± 3.3	41.7 ± 1.5
	OK-432	44.6 ± 3.0	37.0 ± 0.4	43.0 ± 1.5	42.5 ± 0.7

Effector cells were treated for 18 hours with a) RPMI-CS or b) 0.2 u.ml^{-1} OK-432. Natural cytotoxicity for K562, c) Effector:target = 20:1, d) Antibody-dependent cellular cytotoxicity for HRBC sensitized with anti-D at final dilutions 1/800, 1/1600, 1/3200. Effector: target = 1:2.

fluence, OK-432 induced levels of cytotoxicity of comparable magnitude to SEA.

Effect of OK-432 on PBL-NK and ADCC: In concordance with previous data,[6] there was no correlation between NK and K cell activities measured against the respective targets (Table 3). However, whereas OK-432 consistently enhanced anti-K562 activity, under identical pretreatment conditions, the agent was without effect on K cell ADCC.

Discussion

These data establish that, in common with other immunomodulators such as IFN, SEA and lymphokines, OK-432 has a marked enhancing effect on PBL-NK which is consistently demonstrable against both sensitive and resistant clones of the parental erythroleukemic cell line K562. Significantly, this effect also extends to extravascular NK upon which other immunomodulators (with the notable exception of IFN-α on tonsillar lymphocytes)[1] have generally proved to be active. Although basal levels of NK activity are generally low in comparison with those in peripheral blood, the deficit is not an absolute property of extravascular lymphoid tissue. Thus, the identification of macromolecules, which augment pre-existing or induce de novo natural cytotoxicity in various compartments of the lymphon, may have important biological implications for tumor-host interactions.

The mediators of the enhancement of extravascular NK activity by SEA and lymphokines from polyclonally-activated lymphocytes have yet to be defined in molecular terms. IFN-γ and/or IL-2 are likely candidates largely because partially purified preparations of both these molecular species augment PBL-NK.[10,11] Since OK-432 also induces IFN-γ and IL-2 in human PBL,[7] (unpublished data from the laboratory) it is possible that enhancement of NK function by this agent occurs secondary to production of these factors. While this interpretation is consistent with our (unpublished) observations that PBL-NK enhancement can be mediated by soluble factors generated by OK-432 in PBL, a direct effect of the streptococcal immunopotentiator on NK cells which is independent of lymphokine production, cannot presently be excluded.

The lack of K cell stimulation by OK-432 emphasizes an apparent distinction between K and NK activation previously documented using IFN-α.[4] Since recent evidence, based on phenotypic analysis and cloning of NK/K cells, has confirmed their virtual identity,[12] the differential responsiveness of NK and K cell activities to OK-432 appears to be primarily functional. However, this observation should be interpreted with the awareness that the conditions for K cell enhancement by OK-432 may differ from those which are optimal for NK enhancement. If immunopotentiation by OK-432 is indeed mediated primarily by lymphokines, then some enhancement of K cell function might be expected, since both SEA and supernatants rich in IL-2 are effective, albeit to a variable degree, in this capacity (unpublished observations). The fact that enhancement of ADCC by these factors is less marked than that of NK suggests that, unlike the latter function, the ADCC capability of K cells in their native state is nearly maximal.

References

1. Kimber, I. and Moore, M. (1983): Naturally cytotoxic tonsillar lymphocytes: A manifestation of heterogeneity among human NK cells. *Scand. J. Immunol., 17,* 29.
2. Kimber, I., Moore, M., Howell, A. and Wilkinson, M.J.S. (1983a): Nature and inducible levels of natural cytotoxicity in lymph nodes draining mammary carcinoma. *Cancer Immunol. Immunother., 15,* 32.
3. Moore, M. and Vose, B.M. (1981): Extravascular natural cytotoxicity in man: Anti-K562 activity of lymph node and tumor-infiltrating lymphocytes. *Int. J. Cancer, 27,* 265.
4. Kimber, I. and Moore, M. (1981): Selective enhancement of human mononuclear leukocyte cytotoxic function by interferon. *Scand. J. Immunol., 13,* 375.
5. Langford, M.P., Stanton, G.J. and Johnson, H.M. (1978): Biological effects of staphylococcal enterotoxin A on peripheral lymphocytes. *Infect. Immun., 22,* 62.
6. Kimber, I., Bakacs, T. and Moore, M. (1983b): Regulation of natural and antibody-dependent cellular cytotoxicity by Staphylococcal enterotoxin A. *Clin. Exp. Immunol., 54,* 39.
7. Wagasuki, H., Kasahara, T., Minato, N., Hamuro, J., Miyata, M. and Morioka, Y. (1982): In vitro potentiation of human natural killer cell activity by a streptococcal preparation, OK-432: Interferon and interleukin-2 participation in the stimulation with OK-432. *J. Nat. Cancer Inst., 69,* 807.
8. Moore, M. and Potter, M.R. (1980): Enhancement of human natural cell-mediated cytotoxicity by interferon. *Br. J. Cancer, 41,* 378.
9. Kimber, I., Moore, M. and Roberts, K. (1983c): Variance in resistance to natural and antibody-dependent cellular cytotoxicity and to complement-mediated lysis amongst K562 lines. *Int. J. Cancer, 32,* 219.
10. Claeys, H., van Damme, J., DeLey, M., Vermylen, C. and Billiau, A. (1982): Activation of natural cytotoxicity by human peripheral blood mononuclear cells by interferon: A kinetic study and comparison of different interferon types. *Br. J. Haematol., 50,* 85.
11. Gerard, J.P., Bertoglio, J. and Jacubovich, R. (1982): Human interleukin-2 increases the activity of lymphocytes naturally cytotoxic against leukemic and melanoma cell lines. In: *Current Concepts in Human Immunology and Cancer Immunomodulation.* pp.327. Editors: B. Serrou, C. Rosenfeld, J.C. Daniels and J.P. Saunders. Developments in Immunology, Vol.17, Elsevier Biomedical, Amsterdam.
12. Perussia, B., Starr, S., Abraham, S., Fanning, V. and Trinchieri, G. (1983): Human natural killer cells analyzed by B73.1, a monoclonal antibody blocking FcR functions. I. Characterization of the lymphocyte subset reactive with B73.1 *J. Immunol., 130,* 2133.

Lymphokines induction by streptococcal preparation OK-432 (picibanil in mice: Characterization of interleukin 1 (IL-1), interleukin 2 (IL-2) and natural killer cell activating factor (NKAF)

OSAMU ICHIMURA[1], SEIKICHI SUZUKI[1], YUTAKA SUGAWARA[1] and TOSHIAKI OSAWA[2]

[1]*Research Laboratories I, Chugai Pharmaceutical Co., Ltd., Tokyo and* [2]*Division of Chemical Toxicology and Immunochemistry, Faculty of Pharmaceutical Sciences, University of Tokyo, Tokyo, Japan*

Introduction

The bacterial immunopotentiator OK-432 has been an object of great interest because of its potential value in tumor therapy.[1,2] Recently, the so-called lymphokine cascade reaction has widely been accepted as a part of the process of cytotoxic T lymphocyte (CTL) induction, which involves not only cellular membrane interactions and antigen-presentation events, but also a series of differentiation from pre-CTL to functional CTL, mediated by macrophage-derived interleukin 1 (IL-1), helper T cell-derived interleukin 2 (IL-2) and interferon gamma (IFNγ).[3] CTL are believed to mediate the direct destruction of tumor cells in vivo: for example, much evidence has been reported for in vivo protection against syngeneic tumor cells by CTL.[4,5,6] Although OK-432 is known to promote both the induction of CTL against certain syngeneic tumor cells[7] and the induction of IFNγ[8,9] neither the effect of OK-432 administration on IL-1 and IL-2 induction, nor the biochemical properties of OK-432-induced IL-1 and IL-2 have been reported.

Natural killer (NK) cells possess cytotoxic activity against a variety of tumor cells without any presensitization.[10] There is strong evidence that NK cells play an important role in preventing in vivo tumor growth[11] and the metastasis of transplantable tumors.[12,13] In addition, NK cells have the ability to kill freshly isolated autologous tumor cells.[14] OK-432 augments NK cell activity in both humans[15] and mice.[16] However, the nature of the soluble factor most responsible for NK cell activation by OK-432 still remains in question. With these problems in mind, we investigated the culture supernatant of splenocytes and peritoneal exudate cells from OK-432-stimulated mice. As we report here, OK-432 administration augmented both IL-1 and IL-2 production under certain conditions. Furthermore, we found that a new kind of soluble factor termed "NK cell activating factor" (NKAF) plays an essential role in NK cell augmentation by OK-432.

Materials and methods

Mice and tumor cells

Six- to 10-week-old BALB/c female mice were obtained from Charles River Japan Inc. (Atsugi, Japan). YAC-1 lymphoma cells were used as NK target cells and L929 cells were used for the IFN assay. YAC-1 cells were maintained in RPMI 1640 medium (GIBCO, Grand Island, N.Y.) supplemented with 10% heat-inactivated fetal calf serum (FCS, GIBCO) and 60 μg/ml kanamycin (Meiji Seika, Co., Ltd., Tokyo). L929 cells were cultured in minimum essential medium (MEM, Nissui Co., Ltd., Tokyo) supplemented with 5% FCS.

Stimulants

OK-432, a penicillin- and heat-treated, lyophilized preparation of the low virulence Su strain of *Streptococcus pyogenes* (Chugai Pharmaceutical Co., Ltd., Tokyo, Japan), with a KE (Klinische Einheit) unit corresponding to 0.1 mg dried streptococci, was suspended in physiological saline for in vivo administration and in RPMI 1640 medium for in vitro use. Concanavalin A (Con A) was purchased from Sigma Chemical Company (Saint Louis, MO). Lipopolysaccharide (LPS, *E. coli* 055:B5) was obtained from Difco Laboratories (Detroit, MI). Phytohemagglutinin (PHA) was purchased from Wellcome Research Laboratories (Beckenham, U.K.).

Protein assay

Proteins were assayed by the dye-binding method of Bradford,[17] using a Bio-Rad protein assay kit (Bio-Rad Laboratories, Richmond, CA).

Induction of IL-1

PEC were collected from the peritoneal cavity of three mice and washed once with MEM. Washed cells were then suspended in RPMI 1640 containing 10% FCS medium (10% FCS-RPMI) at a concentration of 2 x 10^6 cells/ml. An aliquot (200 μl) of cell suspension was placed in each well of a 96-well U-shape microplate (Limbro Scientific Inc., Hamden, CT). After three hours of incubation at 37°C in humidified air containing 5%

CO_2, nonadherent cells were removed and 1% FCS-RPMI medium (200 μl/well) containing OK-432 or LPS at an appropriate concentration was added. Incubation was continued for 24 hours. Each supernatant was collected by centrifugation at 220 xg for five minutes and then assayed for IL-1 activity.

Determination of IL-1 activity

IL-1 activity was determined by the method of Mizel et al.[18] Briefly, fresh thymocytes of BALB/c mice were suspended in 5% FCS-RPMI medium supplemented with 5 x 10^{-5} M 2-mercaptoethanol (2ME) at a concentration of 1.5 x 10^{7} cells/ml. Then 100 μl of cell suspension was cultured as before with 100 μl of PEC supernatant in the presence of a suboptimal amount of phytohaemagglutinin (PHA, 1 μg/ml) for three days. Microcultures were incubated with 1.0 μCi ^{3}H-thymidine for the last four hours and were harvested on glass fiber filters by using the Labo Mash automatic cell harvester (Labo Science, Tokyo, Japan). Incorporation of radioactivity was determined by scintillation counting in a toluene base scintillator. IL-1 activity was expressed as mean incorporated cpm $\pm$ standard deviation of the triplicate assay.

Induction of IL-2

Spleen cell suspensions were prepared by pressing the tissue through a fine mesh screen into MEM and washing three times with MEM. Then the cell concentration was adjusted to 1 x 10^{7} cells/ml in 1% FCS-RPMI medium containing 5 x 10^{-5} M 2ME. An aliquot (1 ml) of cell suspension was placed into each well of a 24-well multiplate (Nunc. Inter Med., Denmark), and incubated with OK-432 or Con A at an appropriate concentration for 24 hours. After incubation, each supernatant was collected by centrifugation at 220 xg for five minutes and assayed for IL-2 activity.

Determination of IL-2 activity

IL-2 activity was assayed by the proliferation of IL-2 dependent killer T cell line Clone 902. These indicator cells were established in our laboratories from one-way mixed lymphocyte culture. Briefly, after 10 days, responder spleen cells of A/J mice (H-2^{a}, immunized with stimulator cells from C57BL/6 (H-2^{b}) mouse spleen cells (2 x 10^{7} cells/mouse)) were restimulated with stimulator cells treated with mitomycin C (Kyowa Hakko Co., Ltd., Tokyo, Japan). The incubation was at a R:S ratio of 10:1 in 10% FCS-RPMI medium for five days. Then, allogeneic killer T cells thus generated were cloned by the limiting dilution method in the presence of rat IL-2. The "maintaining IL-2" was prepared by the stimulation of rat spleen cells (5 x 10^{6} cells/ml, 5% FCS-RPMI) with Con A (5 μg/ml) for 36 hours. The unfractionated supernatant was used as the IL-2 source. These IL-2 dependent cells had been maintained over six months in the presence of rat IL-2 (25% v/v). An aliquot (180 μl, 1 x 10^4 cell/well) of IL-2 dependent cell suspension, which was washed three times by IL-2 free MEM before the assay, was placed in a 96-well microplate and IL-2 containing samples were added to the microculture at a concentration of 10% (v/v). After 48-hour incubation at 37°C, the incorporation of ^{3}H-thymidine over the last four hours was determined and IL-2 activity expressed as mean incorporated cpm of triplicate assay.

Determination of NKAF activity

Splenocytes of BALB/c mice were suspended in 10% FCS-RPMI medium at a concentration of 1.35 x 10^7 cells/ml. An aliquot (75 μl) of effector cell suspension was placed into a 96-well V-shape microplate (Nunc.). Effector cells were preincubated with NKAF-containing samples (25% v/v) at 37°C for three hours. After preincubation, ^{51}Cr-labeled YAC-1 target cell suspension (100 μl/well) was added to each well. The cells were incubated at 37°C for an additional four hours. Then 100 μl of supernatant was removed and the radioactivity was determined by a gamma counter. Spontaneous release was determined for target cells incubated in the medium alone and total release was determined for 100 μl of target cell suspension. The percentage of specific cytolysis was calculated using the following formula:

$$\text{Percent specific cytolysis} = \frac{\text{Experimental CPM} - \text{Spontaneous CPM}}{\text{Total CPM} - \text{Spontaneous CPM}} \times 100$$

NKAF activity was assayed in triplicate.

Determination of IFN activity

IFN activity was determined by using the 50% plaque reduction method on mouse L929 cells with vesicular stomatitis virus added to the microculture plate as described by Koi et al.[19] IFN activity was expressed in international reference units based on the NIH reference for mouse IFN (NIH No. G-002-904-511). All samples were assayed in duplicate.

Preparation of IL-1-containing culture supernatant for gel filtration

PEC were obtained from 50 mice four days after injection with OK-432 (1 KE/mouse, ip), washed once by MEM and suspended at a concentration of 2 x 10^6 cells/ml in 10% FCS-RPMI medium. Cell suspension was distributed in 30 ml aliquots into 75 cm^2 plastic tissue culture flasks (Corning Glass Works, Corning, NY) and incubated for three hours. Then, nonadherent cells were removed and 1% FCS-RPMI medium (30 ml/flask) containing OK-432 (0.05 KE/ml) was added to the adherent cells. After 24 hours incubation, supernatants were collected by centrifugation at 220 xg for ten minutes. To remove OK-432 particles, an additional centrifugation at 12,000 xg for 30 minutes was performed.

Preparation of IL-2 and NKAF-containing supernatant for gel filtration

The spleen cells of mice, four days after injection with OK-432 (1 KE/mouse, ip), were suspended at a concentration of 1 x 10^7 cells/ml in 1% FCS-RPMI medium containing OK-432 (0.05 KE/ml). After culturing for twenty-four hours, supernatant was collected by centrifugation.

Sephadex G-100 gel filtration

Cell free supernatants were precipitated by 80% ammonium sulfate at 4°C for 24 hours. After centrifugation at 12,000 xg for 30 minutes, the pellets were redissolved in 0.1 M phosphate buffered saline (PBS, pH 7.4) and dialyzed against the same buffer overnight at 4°C, then concentrated 100-fold from the starting supernatant by polyethylene glycol 20,000 (Wako Pure Chemical Ind., Osaka, Japan). For the analysis of IL-1 and IL-2, a small size column (1 x 90 cm) of Sephadex G-100 was used. One milliliter of the concentrated sample was applied to the column and eluted in 1.06 ml fractions at a flow rate of 7.5 - 9.5 ml/hr with 0.1 M PBS (pH 7.4) containing 0.5 M NaCl and 0.02% NaN_3. For the purification of NKAF, a large column (6 x 150 cm) was used. Fifteen milliliters of concentrated materials (44 mg/ml) were applied to the column and eluted with PBS buffer in 14 ml fractions at a flow rate of 57.1 ml/hr. Apparent molecular weight (M.W.) was estimated by comparison with the standard proteins: blue dextran (200 K), bovine serum albumin (BSA, 67 K), ovalbumin (OVA, 45 K), chymotrypsinogen (CHY, 23 K) and ribonuclease A (RIB, 13 K daltons) [(Low Molecular Weight Calibration Kit (Pharmacia Fine Chemicals, Uppsala, Sweden)].

Blue sepharose CL-6B affinity chromatography

Sephadex active NKAF fractions (Fr. 55-65) were collected and purified by affinity chromatography according to the method of Stefanos et al.[20] Briefly, Blue Sepharose CL-6B resin (Pharmacia Fine Chemicals) was washed with 100 column volumes of starting buffer (0.02 M PBS, pH 7.4) and packed into a 12 x 61 mm column. Then, 2 ml of active materials (38 mg/ml) was applied to the column and washed with 10 column volumes of starting buffer E1. After washing, the absorbed materials were eluted with a discontinuous NaCl gradient: second buffer E2 (0.2 M NaCl), third buffer E3 (1.5 M NaCl) and final buffer E4 (50% v/v ethylene glycol in E3 buffer). Flow rate was 2.2 ml per hour and each fraction was 1.06 ml.

Isoelectric focusing-polyacrylamide gel electrophoresis (IEF-PAGE)

The pI of NKAF was determined by IEF-PAGE. The gels (5%, 80 mm) contained 2% ampholytes (pH 3 to 10, Bio Rad Laboratories, Richmond, CA) and were polymerized with riboflavin-5-phosphate (5 x 10^{-6}%), ammonium persulfate (2 x 10^{-4}%) and light for three hours. Samples were dialyzed against distilled water, to which glycerol (15%) and ampholytes (2%) were added. Then, samples (100 μl) were applied to the gels and overlayed first with 100 μl of 5% glycerol and 2% ampholytes and second with upper buffer (0.02 M H_2SO_4). The lower buffer was 1 M NaOH. Gels were electrophoresed at a constant voltage of 200 volts for 24 hours at 4°C, removed sliced into three mm sections, and placed in tubes containing degassed distilled water. The tubes were tightly capped and incubated overnight at 4°C to elute NKAF. The pH of each sample was measured and eluants were dialyzed against distilled water overnight at 4°C. Then all samples were lyophilized, and 300 μl of RPMI 1640 medium were added to each fraction.

IL-2 absorption assay

IL-2 dependent cells were washed three times with IL-2 free-MEM to remove the remaining IL-2. Then the cell pellet (10^4 - 10^7 cells) was incubated in test sample solution (1 ml) at 4°C for four hours, to allow for absorption. The supernatant was removed by centrifugation for five minutes and bioassayed for NKAF and IL-2 activity.

Heat treatment

Samples were incubated at 56°C for 30 or 60 minutes in a water bath to inactivate IFN. After incubation, heat-treated materials were immediately cooled in ice for later use.

Anti-IFN serum

Anti-IFN α/β (NIH No. G024-501-568) was kindly provided by Dr. K. Paucker, Medical College of Pennsylvania, Philadelphia (PA). Anti-IFNγ, a rabbit anti-serum against mouse lymphocyte IFN which is induced by staphylococcal enterotoxin A,[21] was supplied by Dr. M.P. Langford, University of Texas, Galveston, TX.

Acid treatment

The samples were dialyzed against 0.01 M glycine-HCl buffer (pH 2) at 4°C for 24 hours to inactivate IFNγ. To neutralize to a pH of 7.2, an additional dialysis was performed against RPMI medium at 4°C overnight.

Statistical analysis

Student's paired t-test was used to determine the significance of differences between experimental groups.

Results

Augmentation of IL-1 production by OK-432 administration

The action of IL-1 as a signal for the first step in helper T cell activation is well documented.[22] Intraperitoneal (ip) administration of OK-432 induces a number of macrophages, neutrophils and lymphocytes present in the peritoneal cavity.[23] The plastic-adherent population of OK-432-induced PEC was used to produce IL-1. PEC obtained from BALB/c mice 2 to 10 days after injection with OK-432 (1 KE/mouse, ip) were incubated in 10% FCS-RPMI medium at 37°C for three hours. After incubation, non-adherent cells were removed and adherent cells were stimulated with OK-432 (0.05 KE/ml) or LPS (10 μg/ml) for 24 hours. When the IL-1 activity of each culture supernatant was determined by the thymocyte proliferation assay in the presence of a suboptimal dose of PHA (1 μg/ml), significant production of IL-1 in response to the rechallenge of OK-432 was observed in the culture supernatants of day-4 to day-10 PEC. Day-8 PEC produced the maximum amount of IL-1 to OK-432 restimulation. When LPS, a well-known nonspecific IL-1 inducer, was used as an eliciting agent of IL-1 to OK-432-induced PEC, a significant amount of IL-1 was detected in the culture supernatant of day-10 PEC. LPS elicited much less IL-1 from OK-432-induced PEC than did OK-432. We did not detect spontaneous IL-1 production when OK-432-induced PEC were cultured with the medium alone (Fig. 1).

Dose dependent IL-1 production in response to OK-432

To confirm the dose dependency of IL-1 production in response to OK-432 stimulation in vitro, resident macrophages obtained from the peritoneal cavity of untreated mice and day-4 PEC were stimulated with OK-432 (0.005 KE/ml, 0.01 KE/ml, 0.05 KE/ml) or with LPS (1 μg/ml, 5 μg/ml, 10 μg/ml) for 24 hours. As shown in Fig. 2, resident macrophages did not produce

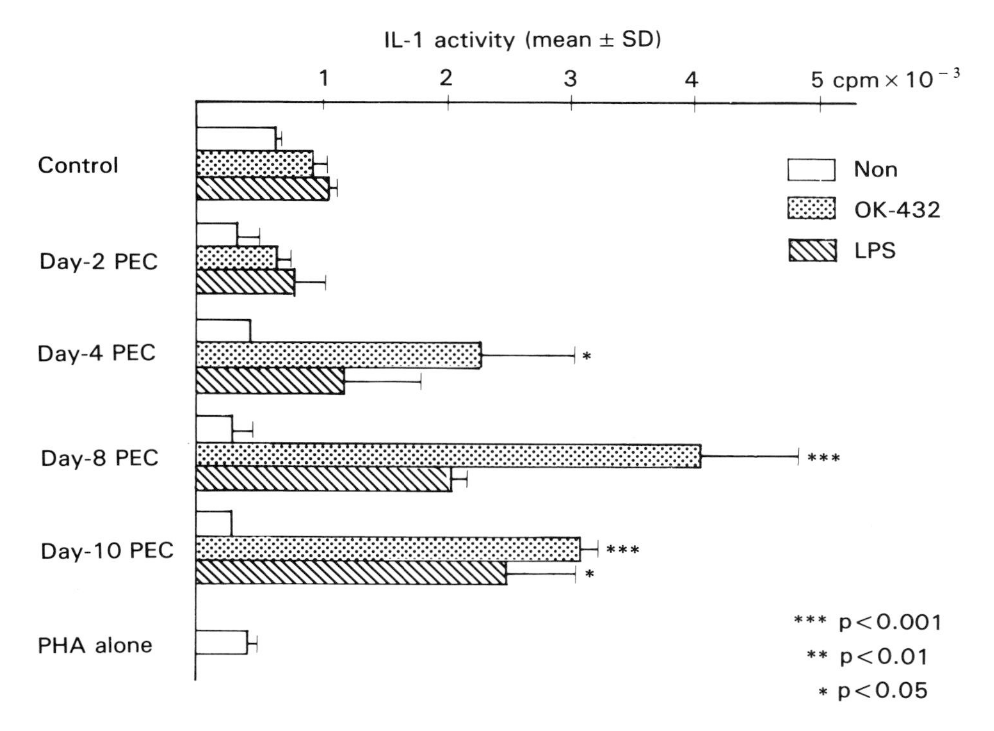

FIGURE 1 *Augmentation of IL-1 production by OK-432 administration.* PEC of BALB/c mice after 2 to 10 days injection with OK-432 (1 KE/mouse, ip) were stimulated with OK-432 (0.05 KE/ml, ▒), LPS (10 μg/ml, ▨) or medium alone (□) for 24 hours. Each supernatant was assayed for IL-1 activity.

any significant amount of IL-1 to the challenge of OK-432 or LPS. In contrast, OK-432-induced PEC showed dose-dependent IL-1 production to the rechallenge of OK-432, but not of LPS.

Sephadex G-100 chromatography of OK-432-induced IL-1

The biological and biochemical properties of IL-1 derived from the macrophage cell line have been established. It is a single molecule which has a molecular weight (M.W.) of 15 K daltons. It is of interest to investigate the molecular weight of OK-432-induced IL-1. The day-4 PEC were stimulated with OK-432 (0.05 KE/ml) for 24 hours in 1% FCS-RPMI medium. The cell-free supernatant, was concentrated 100-fold from starting volume and then the M.W. of OK-432-induced IL-1 were analyzed by Sephadex G-100 chromatography. As shown in Fig. 3, OK-432-induced IL-1 consisted of two major components: high M.W. IL-1 (85 K daltons) and low M.W. IL-1 (15 K daltons). This low M.W. IL-1 coincided with the

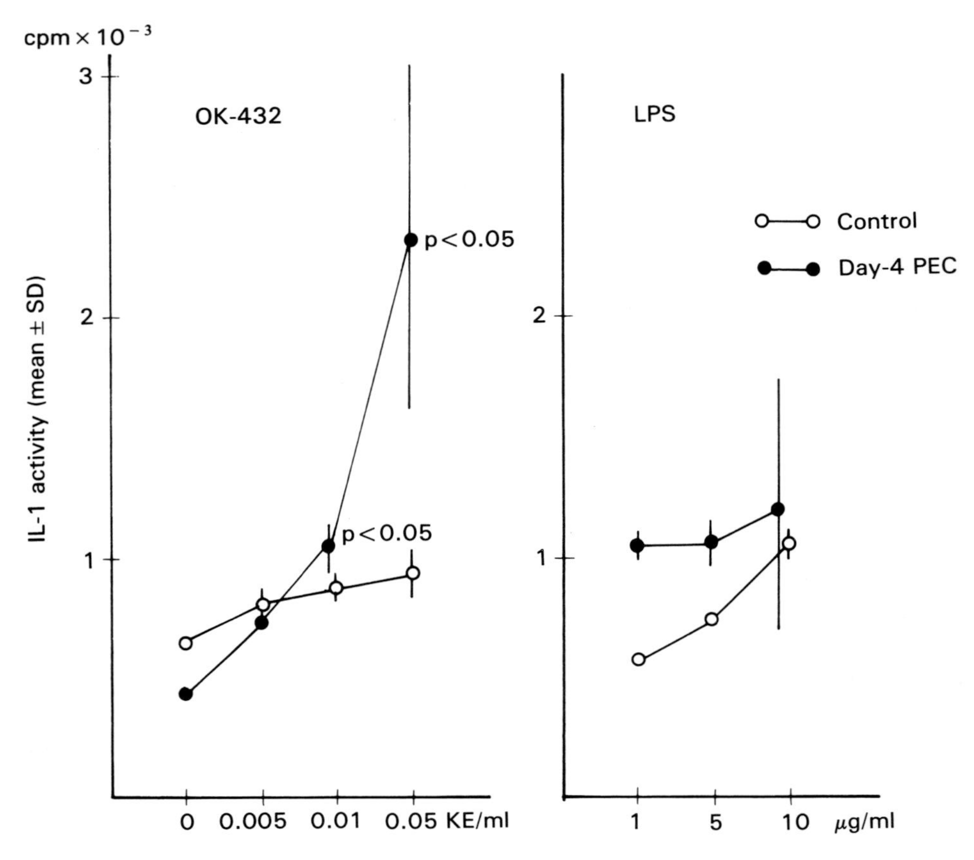

FIGURE 2 *Dose dependent IL-1 production in response to OK-432 stimulation.* Day-4 PEC (●—●) and resident macrophages (○—○) were stimulated with OK-432 (0.005, 0.01, 0.05 KE/ml) or LPS (1, 5, 10 μg/ml) for 24 hours. Each supernatant was assayed for IL-1 activity.

M.W. of IL-1 derived from the macrophage cell line P388D1. Furthermore, the elution profile of OK-432-induced IL-1 correlated with the profile of IL-1 derived from human adherent leukocytes which showed two major peaks (high M.W. 85 K and low M.W. 15 K daltons) on Sephadex G-75 chromatography.[24]

Augmentation of IL-2 production by OK-432 administration

IL-2 is best characterized as a T cell growth factor.[25] Its production can be induced in mouse spleen cells by antigen or mitogen stimulation and it has an important role in CTL induction.[6] To investigate the effect of OK-432 on IL-2 production by splenocytes challenged with OK-432 and Con A in vitro, splenocytes of BALB/c mice 1 to 10 days after ip injection of OK-432 (1 KE/mouse) were suspended in 1% FCS-RPMI medium at

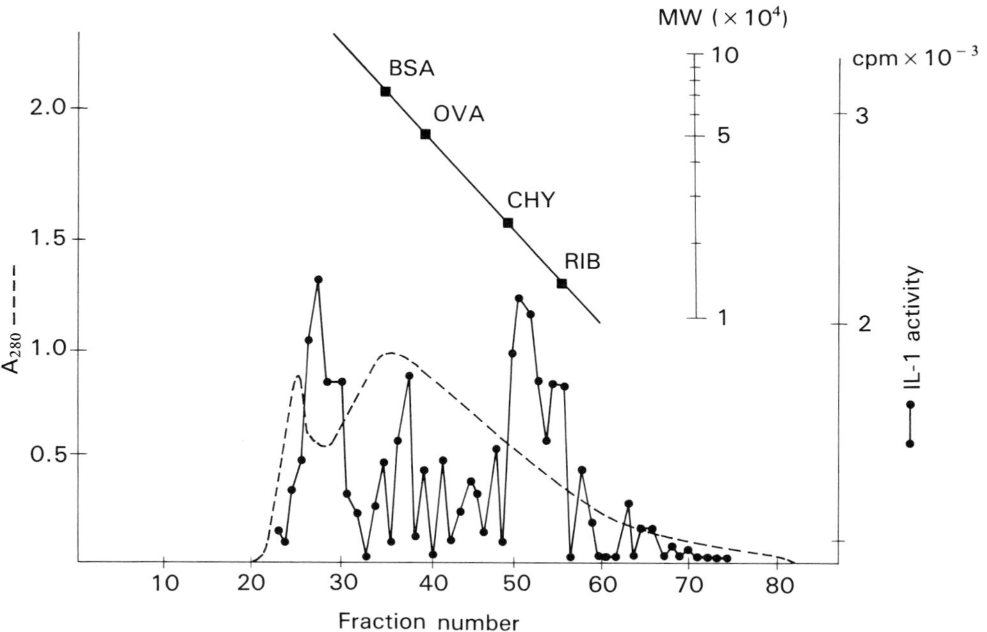

FIGURE 3 *Sephadex G-100 chromatography of OK-432-induced IL-1.* Culture supernatant of day-4 PEC stimulated with OK-432 (0.05 KE/ml) incubated for 24 hours was prepared for chromatography on Sephadex G-100 as described in materials and methods. Each fraction was assayed for IL-1 activity (●—●).

a concentration of 1 x 10^7 cells/ml, stimulated with OK-432 (0.05 KE/ml) or Con A (5 μg/ml) and incubated for 24 hours. When the IL-2 activity of each supernatant was determined by the proliferation assay of the IL-2-dependent cell line, significant IL-2 production in response to OK-432 restimulation was detected in the culture supernatant as early as one day after OK-432 administration. Maximum IL-2 production was observed in the supernatants of day-3 or day-4 splenocytes. When Con A was used as the eliciting agent of IL-2, ip administration of OK-432 gave no significant enhancement of IL-2 production in response. On the contrary, depression of Con A-induced IL-2 production was observed (Fig. 4).

Dose-dependent IL-2 production in response to OK-432

In order to ascertain the dose dependency of IL-2 production in response to the rechallenge of OK-432 in vitro, splenocytes of untreated mice and day-4 splenocytes were stimulated with OK-432 (0.005 KE/ml, 0.01 KE/ml, 0.05 KE/ml) or with Con A (0.5 μg/ml, 1.0 μg/ml, 5.0 μg/ml) for 24 hours. Splenocytes of untreated mice failed to produce a significant amount of IL-2 by OK-432 stimulation, but a significant amount of IL-2 was elicited

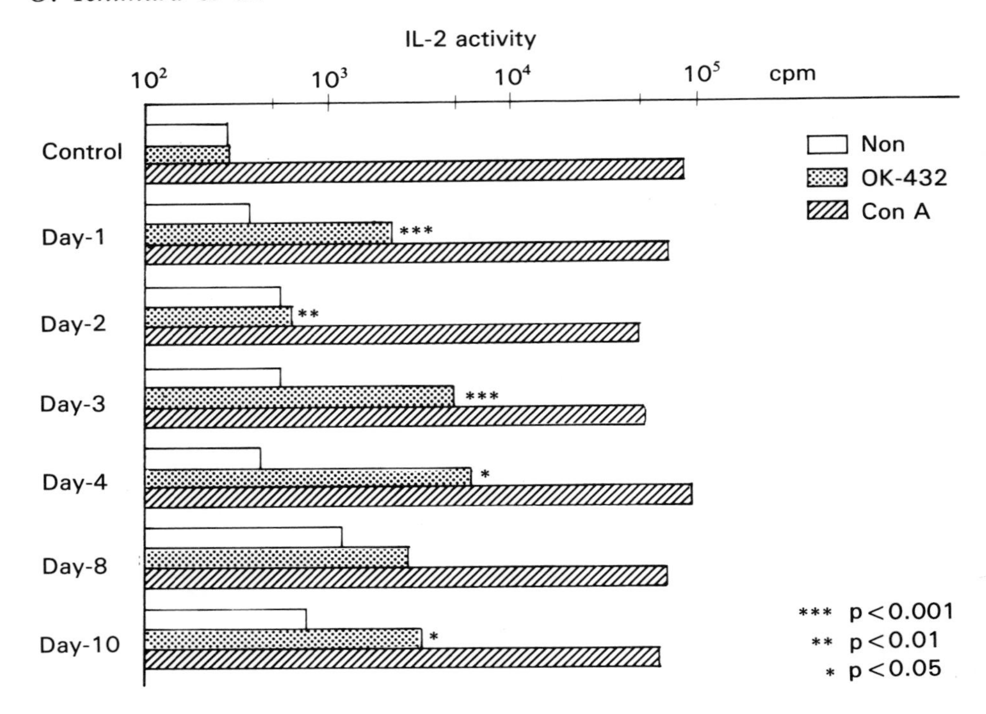

FIGURE 4 *Augmentation of IL-2 production by OK-432 administration.* Spleen cells of BALB/c mice injected with OK-432 (1 KE/mouse, ip) after 1 to 10 days were stimulated with OK-432 (0.05 KE/ml, ▩), Con A (5 μg/ml, ▨) or medium alone (□) for 24 hours. Each supernatant was assayed for IL-2 activity.

by Con A stimulation, in a dose-dependent manner. Interestingly, day-4 splenocytes were able to produce a significant amount of IL-2 to the rechallenge of OK-432 in a dose dependent fashion, however, OK-432 administration did not augment Con A-induced IL-2 production (Fig. 5).

Sephadex G-100 chromatography of OK-432-induced IL-2

Murine IL-2 is a well-defined molecular species, which has a single M.W. of 30 K daltons as measured by gel filtration analysis.[26] To determine the M.W. of OK-432-induced IL-2, culture supernatant of day-4 splenocytes stimulated with OK-432 (0.05 KE/ml) for 24 hours was concentrated 100-fold and chromatographed on Sephadex G-100 column. As shown in Fig. 6, OK-432-induced IL-2 showed a M.W. of approximately 70 K daltons as a single peak, a value quite different from that reported for Con A-induced IL-2[26] and EL-4-derived IL-2 (M.W. 30 K daltons).[27]

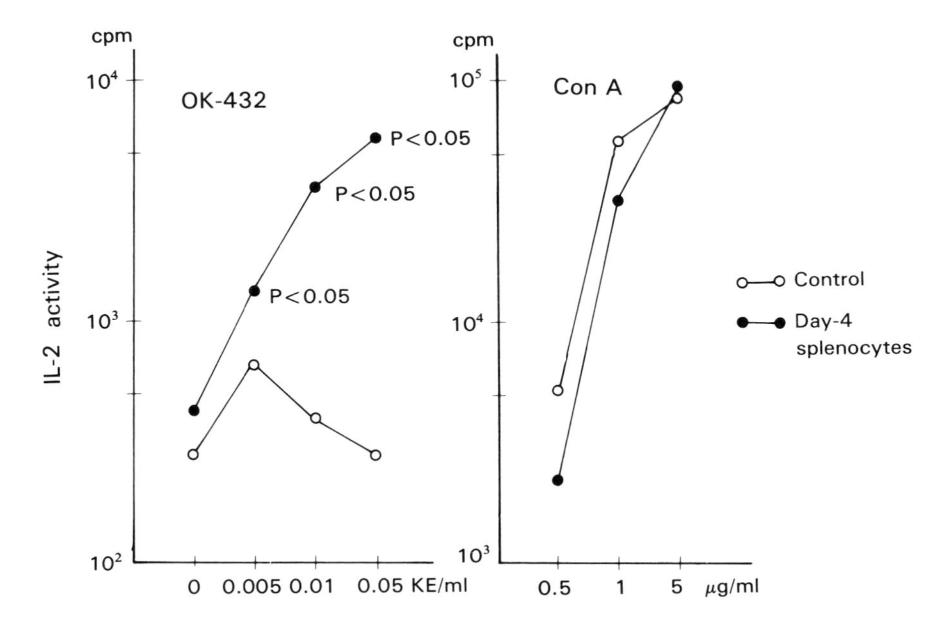

FIGURE 5 *Dose dependent IL-2 production in response to OK-432 stimulation.* Day-4 splenocytes (●—●) and untreated mice splenocytes (○—○) were stimulated with OK-432 (0.005, 0.01, 0.05 KE/ml) or Con A (0.5, 1.0, 5.0 μg/ml) for 24 hours. Each supernatant was assayed for IL-2 activity.

Induction of NKAF from OK-432-stimulated mice spleen cells

Spleen cells of BALB/c mice injected with OK-432 (1 KE/mouse, ip) were isolated 1 to 7 days after injection and stimulated with OK-432 or Con A. Each culture supernatant was assayed for NKAF activity after 24 hour incubation. As shown in Fig. 7, untreated mouse spleen cells produced NKAF, in response to stimulation by OK-432. However, at day-3 to day-5, spleen cells of OK-432-treated mice showed a higher level of NKAF production than spleen cells of the untreated mice. The maximum NKAF production was observed in the supernatant of day-4 spleen cells. In contrast to OK-432 stimulation, Con A failed to elicit higher levels of NK-enhancing substances from mouse spleen cells than those from untreated mouse spleen cells. Although OK-432-priming enhanced spleen cell production of IFN in response to stimulation by both OK-432 and Con A,[33] OK-432-priming did not augment the spleen cells production of NK enhancing substances in response to Con A stimulation.

Sephadex G-100 chromatography of NKAF

In order to investigate the M.W. of OK-432-induced NKAF, culture super-

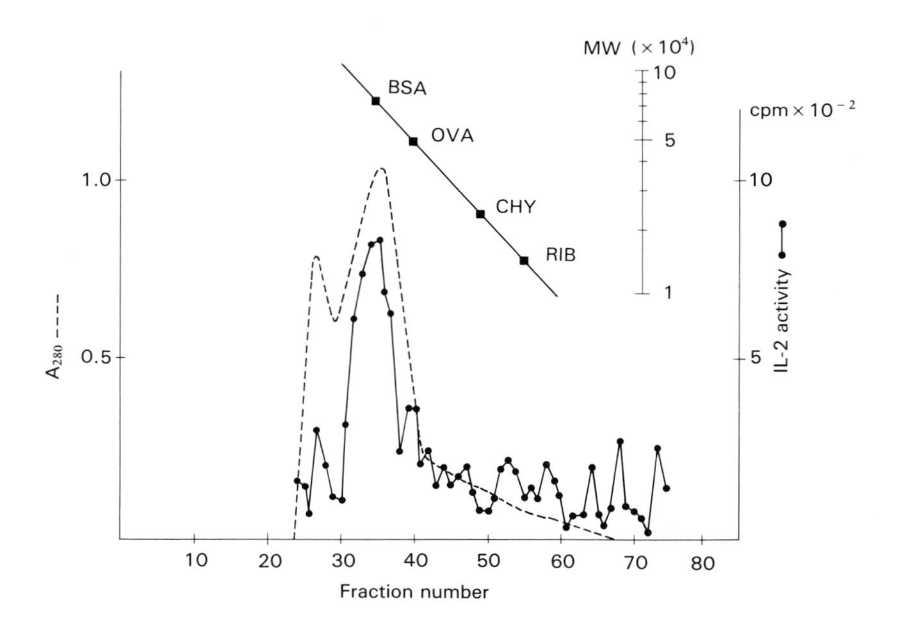

FIGURE 6 *Sephadex G-100 chromatography of OK-432 induced IL-2.* Culture supernatants of day-4 splenocytes stimulated with OK-432 (0.05 KE/ml) incubated for 24 hours were prepared for chromatography on Sephadex G-100 as described in materials and methods. Each fraction was assayed for IL-2 activity (●—●).

natant from day-4 spleen cells stimulated with OK-432 (0.05 KE/ml, 24 hours) was concentrated and chromatographed on a Sephadex G-100 column. A major peak of NKAF was observed at an apparent M.W. of approximately 70 K daltons coinciding with the M.W. of OK-432-induced IL-2. However, OK-432-induced IFN showed molecular heterogeneity: two peaks eluted from void volume to 40,000, at about 80 K and 45 K daltons. From the results of gel filtration, the M.W. of NKAF correlated well with IL-2 but not with IFN (Fig. 8).

Failure of NKAF to be absorbed by IL-2 dependent cells

By Sephadex G-100 chromatography, NKAF and OK-432-induced IL-2 were known to have a closely related M.W. of 70 K daltons. To investigate the relationship NKAF and IL-2, the active NKAF fractions of Sephadex chromatography (fr. 55 - 65) were collected and dialyzed against RPMI medium. Then, the active materials were incubated with IL-2 dependent cells (10^4 to 10^7 cells/ml) at 4°C for four hours. After incubation, each supernatant was assayed for NKAF activity and IL-2 activity. As shown

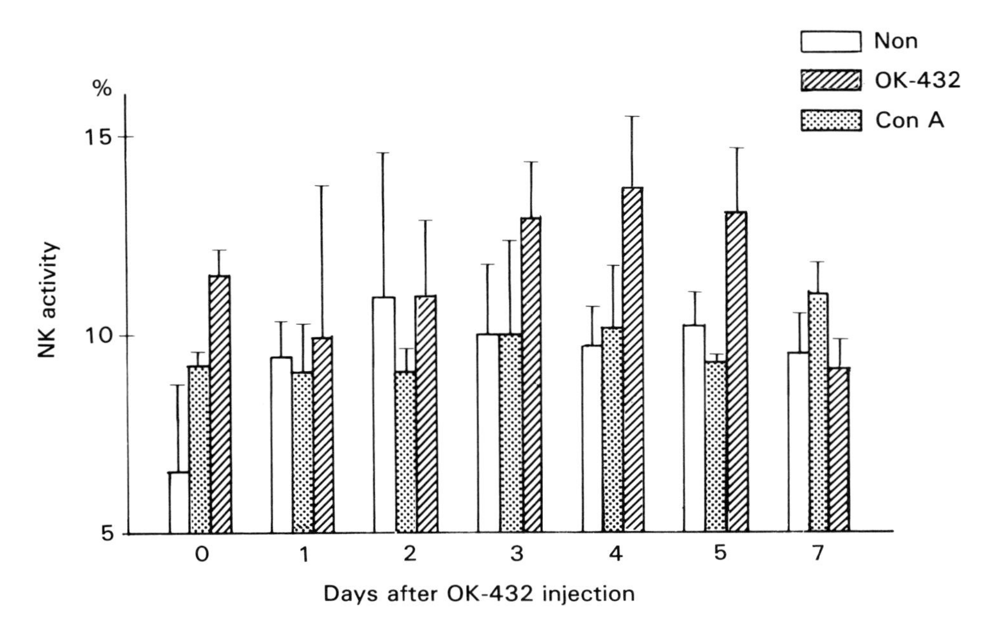

FIGURE 7 *Augmentation of NKAF production by OK-432 administration.* Spleen cells of BALB/c mice given an injection of OK-432 (1 KE/mouse, ip) after 1 to 7 days were stimulated with OK-432 (0.05 KE/ml, ▨), Con A (5 μg/ml, ▩) or medium alone (□) for 24 hours. Each supernatant was assayed for NKAF activity as described in materials and methods.

in Table 1, NKAF activity remained unchanged even after incubation with IL-2 dependent cells. Before IL-2 absorption, the materials did not demonstrate any IL-2 activity in spite of the IL-2 peak fraction obtained by gel filtration. We observed that OK-432-induced IL-2 showed 10 times less activity than Con A-induced IL-2 (Fig. 4) and was labile to concentration and dialysis procedures (unpublished data). Nevertheless, NKAF activity was present in the concentrated materials and was not absorbed by IL-2 dependent cells.

Blue Sepharose CL-6B affinity chromatography of Sephadex active NKAF

IFNγ can be selectively purified by Blue Sepharose affinity chromatography.[20] In order to remove IFN from NKAF containing materials, active NKAF fractions of Sephadex (fr. 55 - 65) were pooled and concentrated (38 mg/ml), dialyzed against starting buffer E1 (0.02 M PBS, pH 7.4) at 4°C overnight, and loaded on an affinity column. As shown in Fig. 9, NKAF and IFN eluted in the same fraction by E3 buffer (1.5 M NaCl containing PBS). IL-2 activity was not observed in any fractions.

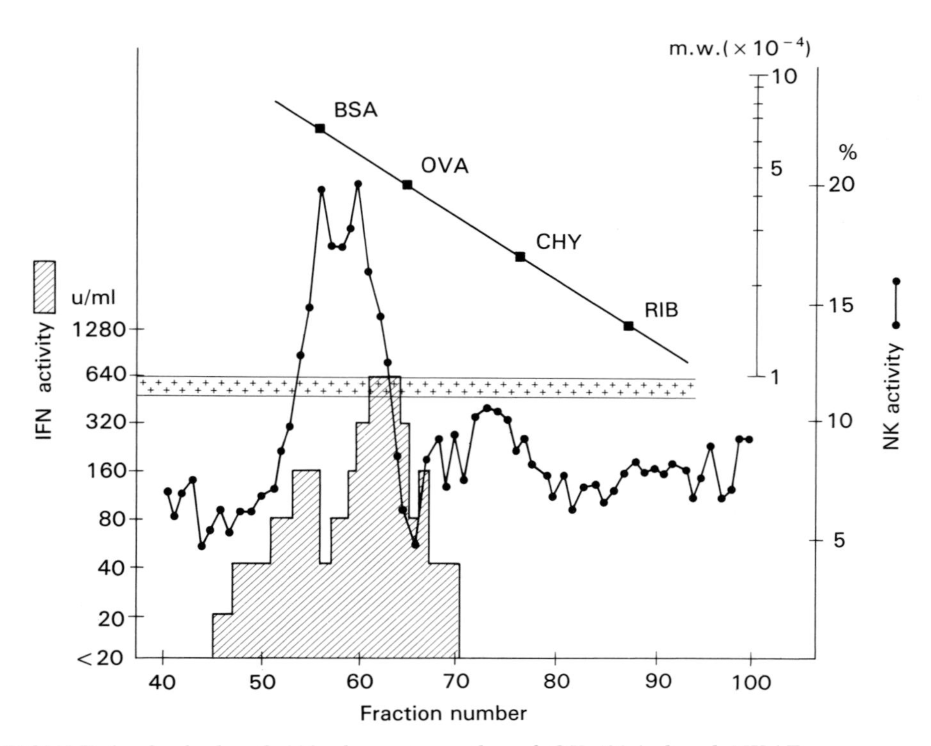

FIGURE 8 *Sephadex G-100 chromatography of OK-432-induced NKAF.* Culture supernatant of day-4 splenocytes stimulated with OK-432 (0.05 KE/ml) for 24 hours was prepared for chromatography on Sephadex G-100. Each fraction was assayed for NKAF activity (●—●) and IFN activity (▨). NK activity stimulated with medium alone was 11.5 ± 1.72 (+++).

TABLE 1 *Failure of NKAF to be absorbed by IL-2-dependent cells*

Absorbed CTLL cell number[c]	Residual NKAF activity[a] ●—● (% specific killing)	Residual IL-2 activity[b] (cpm)
1×10^7	22.2 ± 0.67	94 ± 22
5×10^6	24.6 ± 1.05	54 ± 6
1×10^6	21.4 ± 2.33	59 ± 5
5×10^5	21.1 ± 2.95	59 ± 3
1×10^5	26.6 ± 1.89	76 ± 15
5×10^4	25.3 ± 0.35	70 ± 7
1×10^4	24.6 ± 1.48	84 ± 13
0	20.9 ± 1.92	58 ± 17
Medium alone	7.8 ± 0.99	112 ± 25

Sephadex active NKAF (fraction 55–65) was incubated with IL-2 dependent T cells at 4°C for 4 hours.

a) Each value represents mean activity of triplicate assay.
b) Each value represents mean incorporated cpm ± SD of triplicate assay.
c) Cell-free 10% FCS-RPMI medium was used as control.

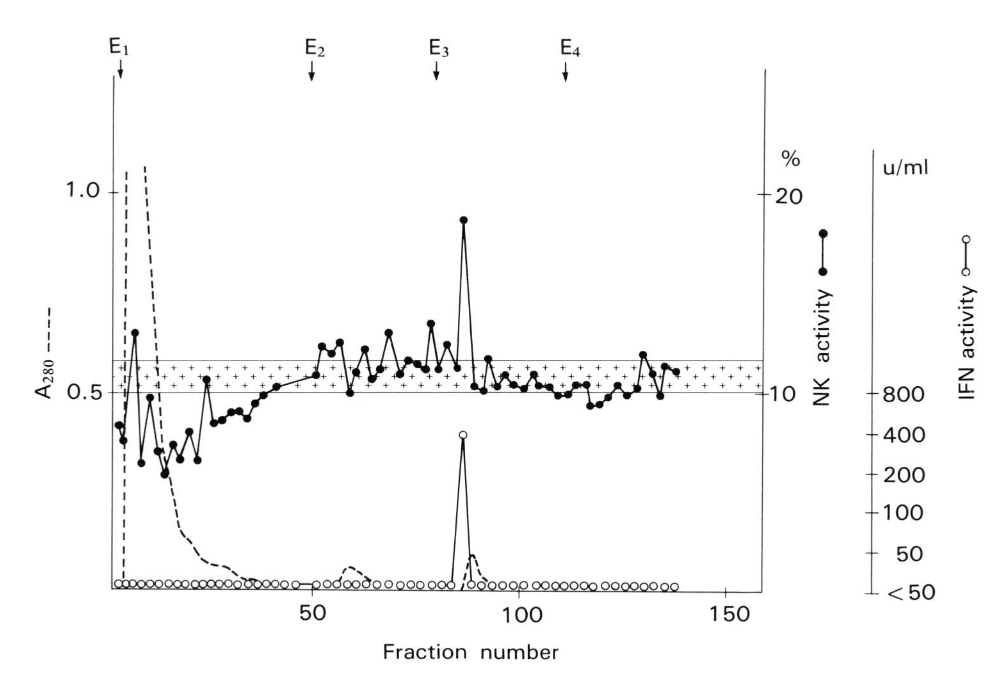

FIGURE 9 *Blue Sepharose affinity chromatography of Sephadex active NKAF.* Sephadex active NKAF fraction (fraction 55 - 65) was prepared for chromatography on Blue Sepharose CL-6B. Absorbed materials was eluted with a discontinuous NaCl gradient. (El buffer, 0.02 M PBS ph 7.4; E2 buffer 0.2 M NaCl PBS; E3 buffer, 1.5 M NaCl PBS; E4 buffer, 50% v/v ethylene glycol in E3 buffer). Each fraction was assayed for NKAF activity (●—●) and IFN activity (○—○). NK cell activity stimulated with medium alone was 10.8 ± 0.7 (+++).

TABLE 2 *Stabilities and anti-IFN serum treatment of affinity-purified NKAF*

Treatment[a)]	Residual NKAF activity[b)] (% specific killing)	Residual IFN activity[c)] (units/ml)
Untreated	11.1 ± 0.36	1280
Heat 56°C 30 min	12.1 ± 0.95	640
60 min	10.4 ± 0.17	640
Acid pH 2, 24 hr	10.4 ± 0.14	320
+ anti-IFN α/β	8.6 ± 0.70	320
+ anti-IFNγ	7.5 ± 1.27	<20
Medium alone	0.2 ± 0.58	—

a) Blue Sepharose active NKAF fraction E3 was treated.
b) Each value represents mean activity of triplicate assay.
c) IFN activity was determined by the plaque reduction method.

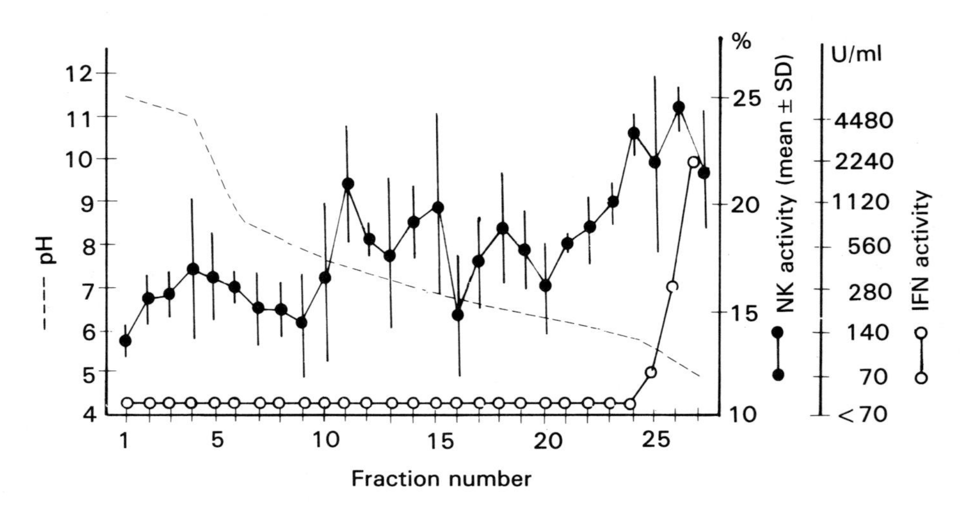

FIGURE 10 *Isoelectric focusing of affinity-purified NKAF.*
Affinity-purified NKAF (fraction E3) was electrophoresed by IEF-PAGE as described in materials and methods. Each fraction was assayed for NKAF activity (●—●) and IFN activity (○—○). NK cell activity stimulated with medium alone was 10.7 ± 1.48.

Stabilities of affinity-purified NKAF and the anti-IFN serum treatment

To compare the physicochemical properties of NKAF and IFN, the affinity-purified NKAF fraction (fraction E3) was treated with heat (56°C, 30 and 60 minutes) and acid (pH 2, 24 hours). As shown in Table 2, NKAF activity remained unchanged after either treatment, however, IFN was sensitive to both heat and acid treatments. Nevertheless, high titers of IFN activity still remained after either acid or heat treatment (320 units/ml and 640 units/ml respectively). It is possible that residual IFN affects NK cell activity. To investigate this possibility, anti-IFN serum was added to the acid-treated materials to neutralize IFN activity. Although anti-IFNγ completely neutralized IFN activity, it failed to abolish NKAF activity. Anti-IFN α/β did not neutralize IFN activity, but reduced NKAF activity to the same extent as anti-IFNγ. Since partial reduction of NKAF activity by anti-IFN serum was not correlated with neutralization of IFN activity, NKAF was distinguishable from IFN by its antigenicity.

Isoelectric focusing (IEF)-PAGE of affinity-purified NKAF

Because IEF possesses a relatively high degree of resolving power in the separation of proteins of similar, but not identical charge, it has been quite useful in comparative studies of the biological activities present in the same cell supernatants. It was of interest to compare the pI of NKAF and IFNγ.

The affinity-purified NKAF fraction was first dialyzed against distilled water, a procedure which did not significantly affect NKAF activity (unpublished data). The dialyzed materials were then electrophoresed for 18 hours at a constant voltage of 200 volts at 4°C. As shown in Fig. 10, NKAF showed charge heterogeneity, with two major peaks (pI 4.0 - 6.5 and pI 6.5 - 8.0). However, IFN had an acidic pI of only 4.0 - 6.0. These data demonstrated that NKAF could be partially separated from IFN by IEF-PAGE.

Discussion

From our results, ip administration of OK-432 augmented a) production of IL-1 by macrophage and b) production of IL-2 by splenocyte in response to rechallenge by OK-432. Since resident macrophages and splenocytes of untreated mice failed to produce a significant amount of IL-1 and IL-2 in response to OK-432 stimulation in vitro, presensitization seemed to be a requisite for OK-432-induced IL-1 and IL-2 production.

OK-432-induced IL-1 showed molecular heterogeneity in gel filtration analysis. However, Farrar et al.[24] reported that the heterogeneity of human adherent leukocyte-derived IL-1 could be resolved into two components (M.W. approximately 85,000 and 15,000). These results correlate well with our observation in the murine system. The low M.W. of OK-432-induced IL-1 coincided with the molecular weight of IL-1 (M.W. 15,000) derived from macrophage cell line $P388D_1$.[22] To our knowledge, the precise biochemical relationship between the two forms of IL-1 has not been investigated. However, it is possible that the high molecular weight form is an aggregate of the low molecular weight form of IL-1 or a complex of low molecular weight IL-1 bound to a carrier molecule. The possibility that the existence of a heterogeneous population of IL-1 producing macrophages resulted in the production of two different forms of IL-1 should be taken into consideration.

OK-432-induced IL-2 had an unique M.W. of 70,000 by gel filtration analysis. According to the previous observation reported by Welte et al.,[28] in the presence of stimulator cells (Daudi cells), human peripheral leukocytes produced another kind of IL-2 which had a different M.W. and pI from IL-2 induced in response to PHA in the absence of stimulator cells. Their findings suggest the possibility that different stimulations may induce different IL-2 molecules from the same cell source. In this sense, the stimulation of mouse spleen cells by OK-432 may have a different effect than stimulation by Con A, because ip administration of OK-432 augments OK-432-induced IL-2 production but not Con A-induced IL-2 production. Furthermore, the M.W. of OK-432-induced IL-2 differed from the M.W. of Con A-induced IL-2. IL-2 can also enhance IFNγ production by T cells.[6] Recently, Saito et al.[33] reported that in vivo OK-432-priming resulted in augmentation of IFN in response to rechallenge by OK-432. These observations strongly suggest that OK-432-induced IL-2 may promote IFNγ production. Taken together, these observations suggest that OK-432 possesses the ability to activate all steps of the macrophage-T cell lymphokine cascade reaction mediated by IL-1, IL-2 and IFNγ. However, it still remains in question whether or not OK-432 can activate the lymphokine cascade reaction in tumor-bearing hosts. Evidence from recent studies support this possibility: we found that OK-432 administration allowed syngeneic CTL generation in tumor-bearing mice (unpublished data). These findings demonstrate that OK-432 can promote syngeneic CTL induction by the activation of the lymphokine cascade reaction, indirectly implicating endogenously produced IL-1, IL-2 and IFNγ induced by OK-432 stimulation, in the promotion of syngeneic CTL generation in vivo.

We found that an IL-2- and IFN-independent pathway in the process of NK cell activation by OK-432 exists, and is mediated by a new kind of soluble factor, termed NKAF. This conclusion was based on the results from the following experiments: 1) NKAF and IL-2 showed similar elution patterns and the same M.W. in gel filtration analysis, while OK-432-induced IFN showed molecular heterogeneity (Fig. 8); 2) IL-2 dependent cells did not absorb NKAF activity (Table 2); 3) affinity-purified IFN was labile to heat (56°C) and acid (pH 2) treatments. In contrast, NKAF was not affected by the above treatments. Moreover, an additional anti-IFN antiserum treatment failed to abolish NKAF activity (Table 2); and 4) NKAF demonstrated charge heterogeneity in IEF-PAGE experiments. Furthermore, a dissociation of NKAF and IFN was observed over the pI range of 6.5 to 8.0 (Fig. 10).

In the human system, Uchida et al.[15] reported IL-2- and IFN-independent NK cell activation by OK-432. Their finding that anti-IFN serum failed to inhibit NK cell activation by OK-432 correlated well with our observations. In contrast to our present results, Wakasugi et al.[29] reported that in culture supernatants of OK-432-stimulated human peripheral lymphocytes, NK-enhancing substances, consisting of IL-2, IFNα and acid-labile IFNγ were induced. These discrepancies may result from differences in species, in the preparation of supernatants from OK-432-stimulated cultures, or in the time of pretreatment of effector cells. We used OK-432-primed mice splenocytes as a source of NKAF and also used a short-term preincubation (3 hours) for NK cell activation. In a short-term preincubation, the production of other NK-enhancing substances such as IFN and IL-2 would be insignificant, as these generally require longer stimulation periods for their induction. However, the possibility still remains that NKAF can enhance the production of other soluble factors, for instance, undetectable amounts of IFN and IL-2 which could in turn activate NK cells, because NK cells themselves can produce IFN.[30]

In the case of athymic nude mice, ip administration of OK-432 markedly enhanced NK cell activity both in the spleen and the peritoneal cavity. Spleen cells from nude mice which had been injected with OK-432 failed to produce a detectable amount of IL-2 in response to OK-432 stimulation in vitro. Nevertheless, NK enhancing substances were observed in the culture supernatants of OK-432 stimulated splenocytes (unpublished data). Saito et al.[9] have reported that OK-432 could induce IFN from spleen cells of nude mice. These findings, coupled with the reported failure of nude mouse lymphoid cells to produce significant amounts of IL-2 in Con A stimulated cultures,[31] have led to speculation that other substances such as IFN or NKAF may have a more important role than IL-2 in NK cell activation in athymic nude mice. Asialo GMl is a well documented NK cell surface marker.[34] When effector cells were treated with anti-asialo GMl serum plus complement prior to incubation with NKAF, both the NK cell activity and the basal level of NK activity were diminished (unpublished data). NKAF failed to augment cellular cytotoxicity against the NK-resistant tumor cell line P815 (unpublished data). These observations coincided with the results of task on the in vivo augmentation of NK cell activity by OK-432, where splenic NK cells activated by ip administration of OK-432 were sensitive to treatment by anti-asialo GMl plus complement and failed to kill P815 target cells (unpublished data).

NKAF showed cytotoxicity against YAC-1 target cells only in the presence of effector cells. No direct cytotoxicity against tumor cells was observed in a four-hour ^{51}Cr release assay (unpublished data). These findings suggest that the NKAF-induced increase of cytotoxicity is only a cell-mediated phenomenon.

In human cancer patients, intrapleural OK-432 administration resulted in an induction and augmentation of effusion NK cell activity, reduction of suppressor cell activity, and reduction or disappearance of effusion tumor cells. Autologous tumor killer cells induced by OK-432 had some NK cell characteristics (e.g. large granular lymphocytes).[32] These clinical findings strongly suggest that NK cell activation is most responsible for the anti-tumor effect of OK-432.

In conclusion, our observations reported here indicate that, under certain conditions, OK-432 augments cellular immune responses mediated by IL-1, IL-2 and NKAF. These findings provide a basis for future studies on the augmentation of cellular immunity against tumor cells by biological response modifiers.

Summary

The present study was aimed at gaining insight into mechanisms by which OK-432 can augment cellular immunity against tumor cells in immunopharmacological aspects. Intraperitoneal (ip) administration of OK-432 (l KE/ mouse) could augment both interleukin-1 (IL-1) and interleukin-2 (IL-2) production to the rechallenge of OK-432 in vitro. Peritoneal exudate cells (PEC) of mice 8 days after injection with OK-432 showed maximum IL-1 production to OK-432 stimulation. OK-432-induced IL-1 consisted of two molecular weight species (85 K and 15 K daltons) on Sephadex G-100 chromatography.

Splenocytes of mice 4 days after injection with OK-432 demonstrated maximum IL-2 production to the rechallenge of OK-432, however, OK-432 administration failed to enhance Con A-induced IL-2 production. In gel filtration analysis, OK-432-induced IL-2 had a distinct molecular weight (approximately 70 K daltons) compared to Con A-induced IL-2.

A new kind of soluble factor, termed natural killer cell activating factor (NKAF) was observed in the culture supernatant of OK-432-restimulated splenocytes, which had a molecular weight of 70 K daltons and which was not absorbed by IL-2 dependent T cells. On Blue Sepharose chromatography, NKAF was co-purified with interferon γ (IFNγ), however, affinity-purified NKAF was stable to acid (pH 2, 24 hour) and heat (56°C, 60 min) treatments. Moreover, NKAF activity was not abolished by anti-IFNγ and anti-IFN α/β antiserum treatments. A dissociation of NKAF and IFN was detected in the pI range of 6.5 to 8.0 in isoelectric focusing electrophoresis. These results showed that OK-432-induced augmentation of cellular immunity against tumor cells might be due to the activation of the so-called lymphokine cascade reaction mediated by IL-1 and IL-2. In addition, NKAF might play an essential role in OK-432-induced NK cell activation.

Acknowledgment

We thank Dr. N. Ishida for kindly supplying antiserum against mouse IFN. We also wish to thank Dr. M. Saito for his technical advice and Dr. A. Uchida for his helpful suggestions.

References

1. Uchida, A. and Hoshino, T. (1980): Clinical studies on cell-mediated immunity in patients with malignant disease; I. Effectors of immunotherapy with OK-432 on lymphocyte subpopulation and phytomitogen responsiveness in vitro. *Cancer, 45,* 476.
2. Torisu, M. et al. (1983): New approach to management of malignant ascites with a streptococcal preparation, OK-432. I. Improvement of host immunity and prolongation of survival. *Surgery, 93,* 357.
3. Farrar, J.J. et at. (1982): The biochemistry, biology and role of interleukin 2 in the induction of cytotoxic T cell and antibody-forming B cell response. *Immunol. Rev., 63,* 129.
4. Gorczynski, R.M. (1974): Evidence for in vivo protection against murine-sarcoma virus-induced tumors by T lymphocytes from immune animals. *J. Immunol., 112,* 533.
5. Shimizu, K. and Shen, F.W. (1979): Role of different T cell sets in the rejection of syngeneic chemically induced tumors. *J. Immunol., 122,* 1162.

6. Bhan, A.K. et al. (1981): The role of T cell sets in the rejection of a methylcholanthrene-induced sarcoma (S 1509a) in syngeneic mice. *A.J.P.,102,* 20.
7. Hojo, H. and Hoshimoto, Y. (1981): Cytotoxic cells induced in tumor bearing rats by a streptococcal preparation OK-432. *Gann, 72,* 692.
8. Matsubara, S., Suzuki, F. and Ishida, N. (1979): Induction of immune interferon in mice treated with a bacterial immunopotentiator OK-432. *Cancer Immunol. Immunother., 6,* 41.
9. Saito, M. et al. (1982): Induction of interferonγ in mouse spleen cells by OK-432, a preparation of Streptococcus pyogenes. *Cell. Immunol., 68,* 187.
10. Herberman, R.B. et al. (1979): Natural killer cells: Characteristics and regulation of activity. *Immunol. Rev., 38,* 70.
11. Habu, S. et al. (1981): In vivo effect of anti-asialo GMl: I. Reduction of NK activity and enhancement of transplanted tumor growth in nude mice. *J. Immunol., 127,* 34.
12. Hanna, N. (1980): Expression of metastatic potential of tumor cells in young nude mice is correlated with low level of natural killer cell-mediated cytotoxicity. *Int. J. Cancer, 26,* 675.
13. Talmadge, J., Meyers, K., Prieur, D. and Starkey, J. (1980): Role of NK cells in tumor growth and metastasis in beige mice. *Nature (Lond.), 284,* 622.
14. Uchida, A. and Micksche, M. (1983): Lysis of fresh human tumor cells by autologous large granular lymphocytes from peripheral blood and pleural effusions. *Int. J. Cancer, 32,* 37.
15. Uchida, A. and Micksche, M. (1981): In vitro augmentation of natural killing activity by OK-432. *Int. J. Immunopharmacol., 3,* 365.
16. Oshimi, K., Kano, S., Takaku, F. and Okumura, K. (1980): Augmentation of mouse natural killer cell activity by a streptococcal preparation, OK-432. *J. Natl. Cancer Inst., 65,* 1265.
17. Bradford, M.M. (1976): A rapid and sensitive method for the quantitation of microgram quantities of protein utilizing the principle of protein-dye binding. *Anal. Biochem.,* 72, 284.
18. Mizel, S.B., Oppenheim, J.J. and Rosenstreich, D.L. (1978): Characterization of lymphocyte-activating factor (LAF) produced by macrophage cell line P388D_1. I. Enhancement of LAF production by activated T-lymphocytes. *J. Immunol., 120,* 1497.
19. Koi, M., Saito, M., Ebina, T. and Ishida, N. (1981): Lactate dehydrogenase elevating agents is responsible for interferon induction and enhancement of natural killer cell activity by inoculation of Ehrlich ascites carcinoma cells into mice. *Microbiol. Immunol., 25,* 565.
20. Stefanos, S., Catinot, L., Wietzerbin, J. and Falcoff, E. (1980): Production of antibodies against mouse immune T (type II) interferon and their neutralizing properties. *J. Gen. Virol., 50,* 225.
21. Langford, M.P. et al. (1981): Antibody to staphylococcal enterotoxin A-induced human immune interferon (IFNγ). *J. Immunol., 126,* 1620.
22. Mizel, S.B. (1982): Interleukin 1 and T cell activation. *Immunol. Rev., 63,* 51.
23. Katano, M. and Torisu, M. (1983): New approach to management of malignant ascites with a streptococcal preparation, OK-432. II. Intraperitoneal inflammatory cell-mediated tumor cell destruction. *Surgery, 93,* 365.
24. Farrar, J.J. and Koopman, W.L. (1979): Characterization of mitogenic factors and their effect on antibody response in vitro. In: *Biology of the lymphokines,* pp. 324. Editors: S., Cohen, E. Pick, and J.J. Oppenheim. Academic Press, New York.

25. Gillis, S. et al. (1982): Molecular characterization of interleukin 2. *Immunol. Rev., 63,* 167.
26. Watson, J. et al. (1979): Biochemical and biological characterization of lymphocyte regulating molecules. I. Purification of a class of murine lymphokines. *J. Exp. Med., 150,* 849.
27. Farrar, J.J., Fuller-Farrar, J. and Simon, P.L. (1979): Thymoma production of T cell growth factor (interleukin 2). *J. Immunol., 125,* 2555.
28. Welte, K. et al. (1982): Purification of human interleukin 2 to apparent homogeneity and its molecular heterogeneity. *J. Exp. Med., 156,* 454.
29. Wakasugi, H. et al. (1982): In vitro potentiation of human natural killer cell activity by a Streptococcal preparation in the stimulation with OK-432. *J. Natl. Cancer Inst., 69,* 807.
30. Handa, K. et al. (1983): Natural killer (NK) cells as a responder to interleukin 2 (IL-2). II. IL-2-induced interferon production. *J. Immunol., 130,* 988.
31. Gillis, S., Union, N.A., Barker, P.E. and Smith, K.A. (1979): The in vitro generation and sustained culture of nude mouse cytotoxic T-lymphocytes. *J. Exp. Med., 149,* 1460.
32. Uchida, A. and Micksche, M. (1983): Intrapleural administration of OK-432 in cancer patients: Activation of NK cells and reduction of suppressor cells. *Int. J. Cancer, 32,* 1.
33. Saito, M. et al. (1983): In vitro production of interferon (IFNγ) by murine spleen cells when different sensitizing agents are used in vivo and in vitro. *Cell. Immunol., 78,* 379.
34. Young, W.W., Hakomori, S., Durdik, J.M. and Henney, C.S. (1980): Identification of ganglio-N-tetrasylceramide as a new cell surface marker for murine natural killer (NK) cells. *J. Immunol., 124,* 199.

Tumor-associated inflammatory cells in ovarian carcinoma: Modulation by OK-432

FRANCESCO COLOTTA[1], ENZO SORESI[2] and ALBERTO MANTOVANI[1]

[1]*Istituto di Ricerche Farmacologiche Mario Negri, Milan and* [2]*Niguarda Hospital, Milan, Italy*

The ability of non-adherent lymphoid cells to kill in vitro tumor cells without overt sensitization has been termed natural killer (NK) activity.[1] The significance of NK cells in vivo has yet to be established. NK activity of lymphoid cells isolated from experimental and human neoplasms have yielded variable results. In some studies, lymphocytes from solid human tumors had little NK activity,[2] while the opposite results were reported in studies of two murine tumors.[2] Unlike tumor cell lines, fresh tumor cells are generally resistant to NK activity.[2] Human ascitic ovarian tumors represent a source of lymphoid cells, macrophages and tumor cells in suspension.[2] The purposes of our study were to evaluate: NK activity of tumor associated lymphocytes (TAL) in ovarian carcinoma ascites, the natural cytotoxicity of effector cells against freshly isolated ovarian tumor cells, and modulation by two agents with reported potentiating effects on NK activity, i.e., β IFN and the streptococcal preparation OK-432.

NK activity of TAL

TAL were isolated from ascitic ovarian carcinoma by stepwise application of discontinuous Ficoll Hypaque gradients.[2] NK activity was measured against the K562 erithroleukemia line[2] in a four- or 20-hour ^{51}Cr release assay.

TAL had low but significant levels of lysis. TAL-NK activity was lower than that of cancer patient PBL, and these were in turn less effective than PBL from normal donors. The defective NK activity of TAL could be attributed either to the absence of effector cells or to the presence of inhibitory cells. To evaluate the second hypothesis, TAL and tumor associated macrophages (TAM) were mixed with autologous PBL in varying ratios.

When the assay was performed immediately, TAM did not exert suppressive activity, whereas TAL did in seven out of 27 patients (inhibition range: 18-60%). Overnight preincubation of PBL with putative inhibitory cells showed no increase in frequency of inhibition by TAL; in contrast a significant inhibition was observed by TAM in five out of eight patients.

A non-specific "crowding" effect appears unlikely. In fact, murine thymocytes and human polymorphs did not inhibit TAL NK activity. Moreover, the low levels of contamination of TAL preparations with tumor cells did not account for suppressive activity, since they were able to suppress NK activity only at concentrations exceeding 10% of effectors. In the attempt to identify tumor associated lymphoid cells with suppressive activity, TAL were passed through a nylon wool column. Both the adherent and the non-adherent fractions were effective in suppression.

To evaluate the possibility of an absence of effector cells, the concentration of LGL, identified as the cells exerting NK activity,[1] in TAL was studied morphologically. Normal and patient PBL had a mean percentage of LGL of 11.2% and 13% respectively, whereas the mean LGL concentration in TAL was 4.6%. Details on this topic are shown in Table 1.

Exposure to IFN[1] and to a streptococcal preparation (OK-432),[3] augments human NK activity. Thus, we evaluated these agents for their ability to increase the defective NK activity of TAL.

As shown in Table 2, both agents (IFN 10^3U/ml and 0.5 KE/ml OK-432 with overnight preincubation at 37°C) were able to augment the impaired NK activity of TAL, with the levels obtained with OK-432 rising somewhat higher than those obtained with IFN. As mentioned above, the low percent-

TABLE 1 *LGL percentages in PBL and TAL of ovarian carcinoma patients*

		Specific lysis (% ± S.D.)	Large granular lymphocytes (% ± S.D.)
Control subjects	(n = 83)	50.1 ± 17.7	11.2 ± 0.5
Patients' blood	(n = 15)	35.9 ± 19.8	13.8 ± 5.1
ascites	(n = 17)	17.4 ± 18.1	4.6 ± 4.7
solid tumor	(n = 7)	9.8 ± 3.2	1.0 ± 0.7

TABLE 2 *NK activity of PBL and TAL of ovarian carcinoma patients*

Effector cells	Specific lysis (% ± S.D.) with		
	Medium	IFN	OK-432
Nornal PBL	34.3 ± 4.0	41.2 ± 2.9	47.4 ± 1.1
Patient's PBL	18.9 ± 0.2	25.6 ± 0.1	33.5 ± 4.0
Patient's TAL	6.5 ± 0.8	not tested	54.7 ± 1.2

A:T = 25:1
Preincubation time: 20 hours.

age of LGL in TAL populations seems to account for the defective NK activity, thus rendering it unlikely that the mechanism of enhancement by OK-432 is an interference with suppressive activity as shown[4] using TAL from malignant pleural effusions.

Lysis of fresh ovarian tumor cells

Unstimulated TAL and PBL from ovarian cancer patients have low or no activity against freshly isolated ovarian carcinoma cells. Generally, levels of lysis did not exceed those occasionally encountered when normal PBL are employed (usually 10% specific lysis at four hours and 15% at 20 hours). Therefore, we were interested in finding out the effects of IFN and OK-432 on lysis against fresh tumor cells. Data are in Table 3.

IFN and OK-432 were able to induce natural cytotoxicity against fresh tumor cells. These effects were best observed in a 20-hour assay. OK-432 boosting was often more effective than IFN-enhancement, both in terms of absolute increase in lysis and in terms of frequency of positive responses. OK-432-stimulated effector cells were able to lyse both autologous and allogeneic carcinomas. As mentioned above, fresh tumor cells from human neoplastic tissue are generally resistant to natural cytotoxicity. Killing of fresh biopsy cells from mainly mesenchimal tumors was seen.[2] This occurred only if allogeneic combinations of PBL and target cells were provided. Similar results were reported by Moore in leukemia patients.[2] Approximately 30% of subjects with various human tumors have PBL cytotoxic to autologous neoplastic cells,[2] but, when histological types of human lung cancer were considered, autologous cytotoxicity was confined to squamous cell carcinoma and to adenocarcinoma.

On the other hand, ovarian carcinoma is relatively resistant to unstimulated

TABLE 3 *Effects of IFN and OK-432 on lysis of fresh ovarian carcinoma cells*

Effector cells	Incubation time	Tumor cells stimulation of lysis/total		Absolute increase in lysis (median with range)	
		with IFN	with OK-432	with IFN	with OK-432
Normal PBL	4 h	5/7	5/10	8.8 (4.0 ± 18.2)	11.7 (9.3 – 19.8)
	20 h	4/7	9/9[a]	11.9 (5.0 ± 16.3)	13.7 (6.3 – 30.3)
Patient PBL	4 h	2/5	2/8	4.3: 11.2	9.6: 11.0
(autologous)	20 h	1/5	6/7[a]	5.5	12.7 (7.1 – 22.9)
Patient TAL	4 h	0/5	1/9	—	7.2
(autologous)	20 h	1/5	5/7[a]	7.1	12.2 (10.4 – 24.1)
Patient TAL	4 h	1/4	1/4	15.8	16.6
(allogeneic)	20 h	3/4	3/4	5.6 (5.0 – 18.8)	18.0 (7.5 – 22.3)

a) $p < 0.05$ (Fisher's exact test) against IFN-boosted cells.

TABLE 4 *Lysis of fresh ovarian carcinoma cells by PBL fractionated by discontinuous Percoll density gradient*

Percoll fractions (% LGL)	Target cells	Specific lysis (% ± S.D.)		
		Medium	IFN	OK-432
Input	K562	28.2 ± 1.4	50.4 ± 1.2	55.4 ± 1.2
(11.3)	ovarian ca cells	4.1 ± 1.2	5.6 ± 1.2	7.3 ± 1.1
II	K562	45.8 ± 1.7	55.1 ± 1.0	68.4 ± 1.7
(70.3)	ovarian ca cells	10.1 ± 0.4	14.6 ± 1.1	21.2 ± 0.6
VI	K562	1.8 ± 0.7	2.2 ± 1.2	3.1 ± 0.4
(0.8)	ovarian ca cells	1.9 ± 0.4	0.4 ± 1.2	1.1 ± 0.9

4 h assay for K562; 20 h assay for fresh tumor cells; A:T = 50:1

effector cells.[2] Our previous findings were confirmed in the limited series of subjects considered in this study, showing that in vitro exposure to OK-432, and, to a lesser extent, to IFN, induced significant levels of lysis of fresh ovarian carcinoma cell by autologous or allogeneic lymphocytes.

Effector cell with natural cytotoxicity against fresh ovarian carcinoma cells

To identify the effector cell with the natural cytotoxicity against fresh ovarian carcinoma, normal PBL were fractioned on a discontinuous Percoll density gradient. As shown in Table 4, the LGL enriched fraction exerted activity against both K562 and fresh ovarian tumor cells, while the LGL-depleted fraction had no activity. This tentatively suggests that LGL may be involved in the lysis of fresh ovarian tumor cells. Similar results on lung carcinoma cells were recently reported.[1] Effector cell involved in natural cytotoxicity against freshly isolated ovarian carcinoma cells needs to be better characterized.

References

1. Timonen, T., Ortaldo, J.R. and Herberman, R.B. (1982): Analysis of natural killer activity of human large granular lymphocytes at a single cell level. In: *NK cells and other natural effector cells.* pp. 9, Editor: R.B. Herberman, Academic Press, New York.
2. Allavena, P., Introna, M., Sessa, C., Mangioni, C. and Mantovani, A. (1982): Interferon effect on cytotoxicity of peripheral blood and tumor-associated lymphocytes against human ovarian carcinoma cells. *JNCI, 68,* 555.
3. Uchida, A. and Micksche, M. (1981): In vitro augmentation of natural killing activity by OK-432. *Int. J. Immunopharmacol., 3,* 365.
4. Uchida, A. and Hoshino, T. (1980): Reduction of suppressor cells in cancer patients treated with OK-432 immunotherapy. *Int. J. Cancer, 26,* 401.

In vivo and in vitro augmentation of natural killing and auto-tumor killing activity by OK-432

ATSUSHI UCHIDA[1], ETSURO YANAGAWA[1] and MICHAEL MICKSCHE[2]

[1]*Division of Immunology, Paterson Laboratories, Christie Hospital and Holt Radium Institute, Manchester, U.K. and* [2]*Institute for Applied and Experimental Oncology, University of Vienna, Vienna, Austria*

Introduction

OK-432, a heat- and penicillin-treated lyophilized powder of the Su strain of *Streptococcus pyogenes*, has been widely used as a potent immunomodulating agent, and has been demonstrated to have antitumor activity both in tumor-bearing animals[1] and in cancer patients.[2,3] Although the therapeutic usefulness of OK-432 has been demonstrated, the mechanism responsible for the antitumor activity of this agent is not fully understood yet. In experimental animal models, OK-432 has been shown to augment macrophage-mediated inhibition of tumor growth in rats,[4] to induce γ-interferon (IFN) in mice,[5] and to enhance natural killer (NK) cell activity of mouse spleen cells.[6] In cancer patients, systemic administration of OK-432 has been reported to cause an increase in both lymphoproliferative responses to mitogens and antigens by a reduction of nonspecific circulating suppressor cells[2,3] and NK cell activity of peripheral blood lymphocytes.[7,8] We have recently reported that local injection of OK-432 in cancer patients results in an enhancement of NK cell activity of tumor-associated lymphocytes.[7,9] In addition, in vitro treatment of lymphocytes with OK-432 has been shown to augment NK cell activity.[10-12]

This in vitro cell-mediated cytotoxicity has been considered one of the expressions of host immune defense mechanisms. In the majority of cancer patient studies on cell-mediated cytotoxicity against tumor cells of spontaneous and activated killer cells, in vitro cultured cell lines have been used as targets. Since in rodent and human experimental systems tumor cells have been demonstrated to acquire the susceptibility to lysis by NK cells through growth in vitro,[13,14] it is difficult to interpret the data on cytotoxicity against cell line targets. In some studies peripheral blood lymphocytes from normal individuals have been shown to lyse tumor cells freshly isolated from the peripheral blood of leukemia patients.[15] Other studies, however, have demonstrated that fresh human tumor cells are relatively resistant to lysis by unstimulated lymphocytes: peripheral blood lymphocytes from less than 30% of cancer patients have expressed cytotoxicity against freshly isolated autologous tumor cells.[16-20] Recently, Vánky et al. have demonstrated that in vitro treatment of peripheral blood lymphocytes with IFN results in an induction of cytotoxic activity against allogeneic, but not against autologous, fresh tumor cells.[21-22] In contrast, IFN-boosted blood and tumor-associated lymphocytes from patients with ascitic ovarian carcinoma have frequently been cytotoxic against autologous fresh tumor cells.[23] In other studies on autologous combinations of effector and target cells, the lysis of fresh tumor cells has been observed with autologous peripheral blood lymphocytes stimulated in vitro by allosensitization,[24] by lectins,[25] and by interleukin 2 (IL-2).[26,27]

We report in this communication that OK-432 is able to induce or augment NK cell activity and cytotoxic activity against autologous fresh tumor cells of peripheral blood and tumor-associated lymphocytes both in vivo and in vitro. The mechanisms responsible for the augmentation of NK and auto-tumor killing activity are also discussed.

In vitro augmentation of NK cell activity by OK-432

As previously reported, in vitro exposure to OK-432 of peripheral blood lymphocytes resulted in an enhancement of NK cell activity (Table 1).[10-12] Blood lymphocytes from normal donors and cancer patients were similarly activated by OK-432 to express augmented NK cell activity. Augmentation of NK cell activity by OK-432 was found to be dose-dependent with a maximum effect at a concentration of 0.5 KE (50 μg OK-432/ml). Kinetic studies have revealed that OK-432-induced enhancement of NK cell activity is evident at as early as 4 hours of preincubation, reaching a peak by 20 hours, and then gradually declining. The manifestation of OK-432-augmented NK cell activity was found to require active cell metabolism, RNA synthesis and protein synthesis, but not DNA synthesis, of effector cells. These requirements were evident since treatment of lymphocytes with OK-432 at 4°C failed to enhance NK cell activity, and actinomycin D and puromycin, but not mitomycin C, inhibited OK-432-augmented NK cell activity.

Removal of monocytes by adherence to serum-coated plastic dishes and Sephadex G10 columns did not abrogate enhancement of NK cell activity by OK-432, suggesting that the augmentation of NK cell activity by OK-432 is independent of the presence of monocytes. However, the possibility that less than 1% monocytes are necessary for OK-432-induced enhancement of NK cell activity cannot be ruled out. Recent reports have demonstrated that human NK cell activity is expressed by a morphological subpopulation of lymphoid cells, termed large granular lymphocytes (LGL).[28,29] LGL consist of approximately 15% peripheral blood lymphocytes, and can be enriched up to more than 90% purity by centrifugation on discontinuous Percoll gradients and subsequent depletion of high-affinity sheep erythrocyte (E)-rosetting cells.[28,29] Fractionation of nylon wool nonadherent lymphocytes on discontinuous Percoll gradients resulted in an enrichment of OK-432-inducible effector cells in low-density fractions 2 and 3, with no OK-432-inducible cytotoxic cells in high-density fractions. These results indicate that the augmentation of NK cell activity by OK-432 is performed by LGL, but not by T lymphocytes.

To determine which type of cells binds OK-432 particles, OK-432 was labeled with fluorescein and incubated either with monocytes, T lymphocytes or LGL. Phase contrast fluorescent microscopic examination disclosed that more than 92% monocytes bound or injested OK-432, whereas only 5% LGL and 5% T lymphocytes bound OK-432 (Table 2). The binding of OK-432 by lymphocytes appears to be nonspecific, suggesting that there is no specific type of cells having receptors for OK-432.

We have previously demonstrated that OK-432 augments NK cell activity independently of IFN induction, since IFN is not detectable in OK-432-stimulated lymphocyte culture supernatants and since anti-IFN-α antibodies did not block the NK-boosting effect of OK-432.[10-12] In contrast, other

TABLE 1 *Augmentation of NK cell activity by OK-432 in vitro*

Dose	dependent (maximum at 50 μg/ml)
Time	dependent (peak at 20 h preincubation)
Temperature	dependent (observed at 37°C but not 4°C)
DNA synthesis	not required
RNA synthesis	required
Protein synthesis	required
IFN	independent
Adherent cells	not required
LGL	involved
T cells	not required

TABLE 2 *Binding of OK-432 by effector cells*

Effector cells	% OK-432 binding cells
Monocytes	92
T lymphocytes	5
LGL	5

Monocytes. T lymphocytes and LGL were incubated with fluorescein-labeled OK-432 for 1 h at 37°C, washed by low-speed centrifugation and examined.

investigators have reported that IFN and IL-2 produced by incubation of lymphocytes with OK-432 are responsible for the augmentation of NK cell activity by OK-432.[30] This discrepancy could be explained by the differences in the lymphocyte activation process by OK-432, since they cultured lymphocytes at a higher concentration of cells in the presence of fetal calf serum (FCS) than we did. Human NK cells have been shown to produce IFN in response to FCS, which could be responsible for enhancement of NK cell activity observed when high concentrations of lymphocytes are cultured in vitro in the presence of FCS.[31] To ascertain whether NK cell activity is enhanced by OK-432 in the absence of FCS, lymphocytes were cultured for 20 hours, either alone or with OK-432, in the presence of either human AB serum or FCS, then washed and tested for cytotoxicity against K562 cells. OK-432 was found to augment NK cell activity in the absence of FCS, indicating that xenogeneic serum components are not required for the augmentation of NK cell activity by OK-432 (Table 3). In addition, no IFN nor IL-2 was detected in the supernatant produced by OK-432-stimulated lymphocyte cultures (unpublished data).

The single cell cytotoxicity assay in agarose has been introduced to detect cytotoxic activity at the single cell level.[32] Application of the single cell level assay has enabled us to examine the effects of OK-432 on NK cells at the single cell level. Overnight pretreatment of LGL with OK-432 resulted in an increase in the frequency of LGL binding to K562 target cells among LGL, and in the number of lytic conjugate forming LGL among LGL/K562 conjugates (Table 4). In contrast, in vitro exposure to IFN of LGL caused an increase in dead conjugated target cells among LGL/K562 conjugates without altering the number of target binding cells. Thus, the frequency of active NK cells was estimated to be higher in OK-432-activated LGL than in IFN-activated LGL. These data are consistent with the findings obtained in the chromium release cytotoxicity assay.[10,11] Furthermore, our preliminary experiments have revealed that OK-432-treated LGL express a more polarized configuration and show stronger motility than untreated

TABLE 3 *Effect of serum on the enhancement of NK cell activity by OK-432*

	% Cytotoxicity	
	Control	OK-432
Lymphocytes cultured in FCS	44.8 ± 5.1	68.2 ± 3.7[a)]
Lymphocytes cultured in human serum	39.2 ± 4.3	63.9 ± 3.5[a)]

Blood lymphocytes (5×10^5/ml) were cultured for 20 h, alone or with OK-432 (50 μg/ml), in either FCS or human serum (10%), then washed and tested for cytotoxicity against K562 at E:T of 20:1.

a) Value is significantly higher than that of untreated lymphocytes at $p < 0.05$.

TABLE 4 *Augmentation of NK cell activity by OK-432 determined in single cell level assay*

Treatment	% Target binding cells	% Dead conjugated targets	% Active killer cells
None	33	40	12.8
OK-432	40	48	18.6
IFN	34	50	16.5
None	41	49	19.2
OK-432	48	58	26.7
IFN	40	55	21.6

LGL were cultured alone or with OK-432 or IFN (1,000U/ml) for 20 h, then washed and tested in a four-hour single cell cytotoxicity assay in agarose.

LGL. Therefore, it seems likely that OK-432 affects the microfilament function of NK cells independently of IFN or IL-2 induction.

Our previous reports have demonstrated that the supernatant produced by OK-432-stimulated lymphocyte cultures (1 x 10^6/ml, 50 μg OK-432/ml) does not contain augmenting factors.[10] However, when blood lymphocytes at a concentration of 1 x 10^7/ml were stimulated in vitro for 20 hours with OK-432 at a dose of 50 μg/ml, the supernatant contained NK augmenting factors (unpublished data). Quite recently, OK-432 has been shown to stimulate mouse spleen cells to produce NK activating factors (NKAF), which are clearly different from IFN and IL-2 (O. Ichimura: personal communication). Taken together, it seems possible that OK-432 augments NK cell activity independently of IFN and IL-2 induction, and that one or more other lymphokines are involved in this augmentation.

It has recently been demonstrated that peripheral blood monocytes, isolated by adherence to autologous serum-coated plastic dishes but not to FCS-coated plastic dishes, can kill NK-sensitive K562 target cells in a four-hour chromium release assay.[33] We have also observed that blood monocytes, isolated from autologous serum-coated dishes, from approximately 30% of normal individuals and cancer patients, express natural cytotoxicity against K562 cells in a four-hour assay (submitted for publication). To examine whether natural cytotoxicity of monocytes is enhanced by OK-432, lymphocytes and monocytes were incubated for 20 hours alone, with OK-432 (50 μg/ml), or with IFN (1,000 U/ml), then washed and tested for cytotoxicity against K562 cells in a four-hour cytotoxicity assay. Enhancement of NK cell activity of blood lymphocytes by OK-432 and IFN was observed in 95% and 80% respectively of cases tested. The level of the augmentation was higher in OK-432-activated lymphocytes than in IFN-boosted lymphocytes (Table 5). In contrast, the lysis of K562 by monocytes was augmented more strongly by IFN than by OK-432. Significant augmentation of monocyte-mediated natural cytotoxicity was observed in 25% of the OK-432 samples

TABLE 5 *Effects of OK-432 on lysis of K562 of blood lymphocytes and monocytes*

Effector cells	% Specific lysis of K562		
	Medium	OK-432	IFN
Lymphocytes	44.8	70.6[a]	59.3[a]
AS-isolated monocytes	10.3	18.4[a]	26.9[a]
FCS-isolated monocytes	2.6	1.2	4.0
Lymphocytes	33.1	54.0[a]	43.3[a]
AS-isolated monocytes	6.6	6.1	18.7[a]
FCS-isolated monocytes	0.3	1.1	0.4

Nonadherent lymphocytes and monocytes isolated by adherence either to autologous serum (AS)- or FCS-coated plastic dishes were incubated alone or with OK-432 (50 Ug/ml) or IFN (1,000 U/ml), for 20 h, then washed and tested for cytotoxicity against K562 at E:T of 20:1.
a) Value is significantly higher than that of controls at $p < 0.05$.

and in 45% of the IFN samples. These results may suggest that OK-432 is a strong activator of NK cells but not of monocytes. The possibility that OK-432-stimulated monocytes produce prostaglandins or other inhibitory substances which inhibit the augmentation of monocyte cytotoxicity by OK-432 cannot be excluded in the present study.

The most potent antitumor activity may logically be expected to be present within or around the site of tumor growth. However, we and others have observed that lymphocytes from solid neoplasms or from pleural effusions have markedly low or no NK cell activity.[34-36] We have also demonstrated that the lack of NK cell activity of effusion lymphocytes is due to the presence of adherent suppressor cells in carcinomatous pleural effusions of cancer patients.[37,38] It seems of importance to know whether OK-432 can augment NK cell activity of tumor-infiltrating or tumor-associated lymphocytes and monocyte/macrophages. As previously reported,[9,11,38] NK cell activity of blood lymphocytes was not augmented by in vitro IFN treatment in the presence of adherent cells from malignant pleural effusions (Table 6). Similarly, effusion mononuclear cells were not activated by IFN. In contrast, OK-432 was found to be able to augment NK cell activity of blood lymphocytes even in the presence of adherent effusion suppressor cells. Furthermore, pleural effusion lymphocytes were activated by OK-432 to express enhanced NK cell activity. On the other hand, the lysis of K562 by effusion monocyte/macrophages, isolated by adherence to autologous serum-coated plastic dishes, was not augmented by either OK-432 or by IFN. Other investigators have also reported that NK cell activity of tumor-associated lymphocytes from ascites ovarian carcinoma is augmented in vitro by OK-432.[39] The enhancement of NK cell activity of pleural effusion lymphocytes may be due in part to the reduction or abrogation of NK suppressive activity of adherent effusion cells, since in vitro overnight treat-

TABLE 6 *In vitro augmentation of effusion NK cell activity by OK-432*

Effector cells	% Cytotoxicity		
	Medium	OK-432	IFN
Blood lymphocytes	35.1	60.3[a)]	51.6[a)]
Blood lymphocytes + Effusion adherent cells	10.8	46.2[a)]	11.9
Effusion lymphocytes	5.8	20.4[a)]	4.4
Effusion adherent cells	3.7	2.6	4.0

Effector cells were incubated alone or with OK-432 or IFN for 20 h, then washed and tested for lysis of K562 at E:T of 20:1.
a) Value is significantly higher than that of controls at $p < 0.05$.

ment of adherent effusion suppressor cells with OK-432 caused adherent effusion cells to be non-suppressive.[9,38] In animal experimental models adherent peritoneal cells from normal mice have been shown to have NK suppressive activity, which could be eliminated by treatment with *Corynebacterium parvum*.[40] Similar mechanisms might be involved in the abrogation of suppressor function in both systems.

It has been demonstrated that NK cell activity of lymph node lymphocytes is relatively low and hardly augmented by IFN.[41] For this reason we examined whether or not OK-432 can augment NK cell activity of lymph node lymphocytes. When lymph node lymphocytes from patients with various cancers were stimulated in vitro with OK-432 for 20 hours, the lymphocytes showed augmented NK cell activity (Table 7). In contrast, in vitro overnight exposure to IFN of lymph node lymphocytes resulted, in most cases, in no enhancement of NK cell activity. In a few cases, IFN enhanced lymph node NK cell activity, but the level was lower than that of OK-432 activated lymph node lymphocytes. In contrast to pleural effusion mononuclear cells, no NK suppressor cells were observed in lymph node cells. These results again suggest that OK-432 enhances NK cell activity of extravascular lymphocytes independently of IFN induction.

In vivo augmentation of NK cell activity by OK-432

Based on the in vitro NK enhancing effect of OK-432, it was used as treatment for cancer patients. For a clinical application of OK-432, it seems important to determine which route of administration of OK-432 is most effective for the boosting of blood NK cell activity in cancer patients. As previously reported,[7,9] a single intravenous or intradermal injection of 1 KE of OK-432 resulted in a rapid, strong augmentation of blood NK cell activity, being detectable on day 1, peaking on day 3 and then returning to base line levels within 7 days (Table 7). In contrast, only a small enhance-

TABLE 7 *Augmentation of blood NK cell activity by systemic administration of OK-432*

Administration route	Cytotoxicity (RCI)				
	Day 0	Day 1	Day 2	Day 3	Day 7
None	1.13	0.87	1.00	1.23	0.77
Intravenous	0.52	2.16[a)]	4.10[a)]	5.77[a)]	1.22[a)]
Intradermal	0.42	1.45[a)]	2.81[a)]	3.55[a)]	0.68
Intramuscular	0.90	0.48	1.22	1.45[a)]	1.10

Cancer patients received either intravenous, intradermal or intramuscular injection of 1 KE of OK-432 on day 0 and monitored for NK cell activity against K562 from day 0 to day 7. Results are expressed as relative cytotoxic index (RCI), calculated as lytic units/10^7 cells of OK-432-treated patients' blood lymphocytes divided by the mean of control untreated subjects' blood lymphocytes determined on 5 independent occasions. Where cytotoxicity indices differed by greater then 2 SD from controls, values are considered significant a).

ment of blood NK cell activity was obtained on day 3 in cancer patients who received an intramuscular injection. These results indicate that the route of administration is an important variable. The enhancement of blood NK cell activity by OK-432 administration is unlikely to be derived from the redistribution of NK cells but may result from the stimulation of lytic function of blood NK cells, since the frequency of LGL among peripheral blood lymphocytes was not altered by the OK-432 administration. No increase in IFN levels was seen in the peripheral blood of patients undergoing OK-432 injection, suggesting that the augmentation of blood NK cell activity by OK-432 therapy is not mediated through IFN. Other investigators have reported that blood NK cell activity is increased by daily intramuscular injections of OK-432 in cancer patients.[42]

Intrapleural or intraperitoneal injections of OK-432 have been shown to cause a reduction or disappearance of effusions and tumor cells in the pleural cavity or peritoneal cavities of cancer patients.[43] To clarify the mechanism responsible for the antitumor activity of intrapleurally injected OK-432, we monitored effusion NK cell activity and NK suppressor cell activity of adherent effusion cells after intrapleural administration of OK-432.[7,9] NK cell activity against K562 was markedly low or absent in pleural effusions of cancer patients before OK-432 therapy (Table 8). Seven days after a single intrapleural injection of 10 KE of OK-432, two non-responder patients, who had no clinical improvement with the OK-432 therapy, still had no NK cell activity in their pleural effusions. The other seven responder patients, who showed a reduction or disappearance of tumor cells in their pleural effusions, had an induction or marked augmentation of effusion NK cell activity on day 7, which was even higher than the blood NK cell activity of normal donors. Furthermore, adherent effusion cells, which previously inhibited the maintenance of functional NK cells and IFN-induced development of active

TABLE 8 *Blood and effusion NK cell activity before and after intrapleural injection of OK-432*

Subjects	Cytotoxicity (LU)			
	Effusion		Blood	
	Day 0	Day 7	Day 0	Day 7
Nonresponder patients (2)[a]	<0.1	<0.1	4.7 ± 1.8	2.8 ± 3.0
Responder patients (7)[b]	0.5 ± 0.3	21.4 ± 4.3[f]	7.3 ± 2.0	10.8 ± 2.8
Responder patients (3)[c]	0.5 ± 0.5	—	8.0 ± 2.5	10.5 ± 2.0
Control patients (8)[d]	9.4 ± 2.1	—	—	—
Control donors (25)[e]	—	12.3 ± 0.7	—	13.0 ± 0.9

Twelve cancer patients with malignant pleural effusions were treated with a single intrapleural injection of 10 KE of OK-432. Blood and effusion NK cell activity was tested before and 7 days after OK-432 injection.

a) Patients showed no reduction of pleural effusions and effusion tumors.
b) Patients showed reduction or disappearance of tumor cells in their effusions.
c) Patients showed a complete disappearance of pleural effusions.
d) Effusion controls from patients with nonmalignant pleural effusions.
e) Blood controls from normal healthy individuals.
f) Value is significantly higher than that of day 0 ($p < 0.05$).

NK cells, lost their NK suppressive activity during seven days of OK-432 treatment (Table 9). It should be noted that the reduction or disappearance of tumor cells in pleural effusions is strongly associated with the induction or augmentation of effusion NK cell activity in patients who received intrapleural injection of OK-432. On the other hand, blood NK cell activity was not consistently modified by the intrapleural OK-432 therapy. These results suggest that at least OK-432-activated tumor-associated NK cells interact in vivo with autologous tumor cells.

In vitro augmentation of auto-tumor killing activity by OK-432

We have recently demonstrated that a minor proportion of human NK cells can kill autologous fresh tumor cells in a short-term assay.[19] Since IFN has been shown not to induce cytotoxic activity against autologous tumor cells,[21,22] it seems of practical importance to examine whether OK-432 induces or augments auto-tumor killing activity of blood and tumor-associated lymphocytes. Tumor cells were isolated from pleural effusions of cancer patients by discontinuous Ficoll-Hypaque centrifugation, then by discontinuous Percoll gradient centrifugation and subsequent depletion of adherent nonmalignant cells, as previously described.[19] Freshly isolated pleural effusion tumor cells were found to be relatively resistant to lysis by unstimulated

TABLE 9 *Reduction of NK suppressor activity of adherent effusion cells by intrapleural injection of OK-432*

Subjects	% NK Suppression	
	Day 0	Day 7
Nonresponder patients	64.5 ± 9.5[a]	47.5 ± 7.5[a]
Responder patients	53.1 ± 5.5[a]	2.8 ± 4.9
Control patients	2.6 ± 5.3	—

Patients with malignant pleural effusions were intrapleurally given 10 KE of OK-432 on day 0. Adherent cells from pleural effusions of the patients were tested for NK suppressor activity after overnight incubation with normal blood lymphocytes.
a) Value is significant ($p < 0.05$).

TABLE 10 *Cytotoxicity against autologous effusion tumor cells of unstimulated and OK-432-activated blood and effusion lymphocytes*

Effector cells	% Cytotoxicity	Positive reaction (%)
Blood		
Unstimulated lymphocytes	4.3 ± 1.0 (0–22)	4/28 (14.3)
OK-432-activated lymphocytes	17.8 ± 2.4 (0–43)[a]	21/28 (75.0)[a]
Effusion		
Unstimulated lymphocytes	4.5 ± 1.2 (0–25)	5/28 (17.9)
OK-432-activated lymphocytes	17.5 ± 2.3 (0–40)[a]	21/25 (75.0)[a]

Blood and effusion lymphocytes were cultured alone or with OK-432 (50 μg/ml) for 20 h, then washed and tested for cytotoxicity against autologous effusion tumor cells in a 4 h chromium release assay at E:T of 40:1. a) Cytotoxicity >8% was considered significant.

lymphocytes (Table 10). Positive reactions were recorded in 14% of the blood lymphocyte and 18% of the effusion lymphocyte samples. To determine optimal conditions for an induction or augmentation of auto-tumor killing activity by OK-432, blood and effusion lymphocytes were incubated with varying concentrations of OK-432 for 20 hours prior to cytotoxicity assays against autologous effusion tumor cells. The maximum induction of auto-tumor killing activity was observed when effector cells were treated with 50 μg OK-432/ml (Table 11). Both blood and effusion lymphocytes were maximumly activated with the dose of OK-432. The same dose of OK-432 was found to augment NK cell activity against K562 cells. After activation with OK-432, an induction of auto-tumor killing activity was recorded in 70.8% of the blood lymphocyte samples and 69.6% of the effusion lymphocyte specimens that initially had no cytotoxicity against autologous tumor cells.[20] When unstimulated lymphocytes already had significant cytotoxicity, their auto-tumor killing activity was augmented in all cases by in vitro

TABLE 11 *OK-432 dose-dependent induction of cytotoxicity against autologous tumor cells*

OK-432 concentrations (μg/ml)	% Cytotoxicity			
	Blood lymphocytes		Effusion lymphocytes	
	Auto-tumor	K562	Auto-tumor	K562
0	4.8	30.5	3.5	8.0
1	2.3	48.6[a]	1.8	20.1[a]
10	8.9[a]	51.4[a]	14.6[a]	29.3[a]
50	20.0[a]	61.4[a]	31.8[a]	34.7[a]
100	10.7[a]	47.1[a]	15.2[a]	21.2[a]

Blood and effusion lymphocytes were cultured alone or with various concentrations of OK-432 for 20 h, then washed and tested for cytotoxicity against autologous effusion tumor cells and K562 cells at E:T of 40:1.
a) Value is significantly higher than that of controls ($p < 0.05$).

exposure to OK-432. Thus, of 28 blood and effusion samples, 75% showed OK-432-induced lysis of autologous fresh tumor cells, whereas only 14% and 18% of unstimulated blood and effusion lymphocytes killed autologous tumor cells (Table 10). OK-432-activated blood and effusion lymphocytes from cancer patients were also capable of killing allogeneic fresh effusion tumor cells (unpublished data). Furthermore, OK-432-boosted blood lymphocytes from normal donors were found to lyse fresh allogeneic effusion tumor cells in a four-hour assay. These results indicate that OK-432-induced lysis of fresh tumor cells is not restricted to cancer patients, and therefore can not be considered as a specific anamnestic response.

Since OK-432-induced enhancement of NK cell activity has been shown to require active cell metabolism and RNA and protein syntheses of effector cells,[10-12] the next experiments were performed to determine the metabolic processes required for the manifestation of OK-432-induced auto-tumor killing activity. Pretreatment of lymphocytes with mitomycin C resulted in no inhibition of unstimulated auto-tumor killing activity nor abrogation of OK-432-induced lysis of autologous tumor cells (Table 12). In contrast, pretreatment with actinomycin D or treatment with puromycin before and during OK-432 activation resulted in abrogation of both unstimulated and OK-432-induced auto-tumor killing activity. These results indicate that RNA and protein syntheses, but not DNA synthesis, of effector cells are required for the manifestation of OK-432-induced lysis of fresh autologous tumor cells. Our findings are in agreement with other observations that proliferation is not necessary for the induction of auto-tumor killing activity by lectins.[25] In contrast, IL-2-induced activation of cytotoxic cells has been reported to be susceptible to irradiation.[26,27]

Several attempts have been made to activate human lymphocytes to kill

TABLE 12 *Effects of metabolic inhibitors on unstimulated and OK-432-induced cytotoxicity against autologous tumor cells*

Incubation with metabolic inhibitors	% Cytotoxicity against autologous tumor			
	Blood lymphocytes		Effusion lymphocytes	
	Control	OK-432	Control	OK-432
Medium	4.0 ± 3.0	20.9 ± 5.1[a]	6.5 ± 2.9	23.2 ± 4.2[a]
Mitomycin C	1.8 ± 2.4	18.0 ± 5.5[a]	3.7 ± 3.4	20.2 ± 2.8[a]
Actinomycin D	1.9 ± 1.3	2.6 ± 1.3	1.4 ± 1.2	4.5 ± 1.1
Puromycin	2.7 ± 0.9	0.0 ± 1.8	0.8 ± 1.3	1.7 ± 1.7

Blood and effusion lymphocytes were incubated for 1 h with medium, mitomycin C (50 μg/ml), actinomycin D (10 μg/ml), or puromycin (10 μg/ml). They were then washed (those in mitomycin or actinomycin) or left unwashed (those in medium or puromycin) and were further incubated alone or with OK-432 (50 μg/ml) for 20 h, then washed and tested for cytotoxicity against autologous effusion tumor cells at E:T of 40:1. Results are expressed as the mean ±SE of 5 different experiments.
a) Value is significantly higher than that of corresponding control cells at $p < 0.05$.

fresh autologous tumor cells. Fresh tumor cells can be killed by autologous lymphocytes grown in medium containing IL-2.[26,27] In vitro exposure to β-IFN causes a low-level of killing of autologous fresh ovarian tumor cells.[23] We, therefore, examined the possibility that OK-432-activated cells produce factors that have enhancing capacities such as those of IL-2 and IFN. Blood and effusion lymphocytes were stimulated in vitro with cell-free supernatants, produced by 20-hour OK-432-stimulated lymphocyte cultures, for 20 hours before they were tested for cytotoxicity against autologous fresh tumor cells. The supernatant failed to induce auto-tumor killing activity (Table 13), while lymphocytes activated with OK-432 were induced to kill autologous tumor cells. Furthermore, treatment of lymphocytes with the doses of IL-2 and IFN that were able to augment NK cell activity caused no induction nor augmentation of auto-tumor killing activity. These results suggest that OK-432 activates lymphocytes cytotoxic to fresh autologous effusion tumor cells independently of IFN and IL-2 induction. Our findings are in keeping with previous reports that short-term in vitro exposure to α-IFN is incapable of activating lymphocytes to lyse autologous tumor cells,[21,22] and that a two- to three-day culture of blood lymphocytes in medium containing IL-2 is necessary for the generation of lymphokine-activated killer cells.[27]

The possibility that OK-432-activated killer cells are identical to lectin-activated killer cells cannot be excluded in the present study. However, the maximum appearance of lectin-activated killer cells has been demonstrated to require three days of culture and to coincide with the maximum appearance of cells with blastoid morphology in the culture,[25] whereas overnight culture with 50 μg OK-432/ml was found to be optimum for the genera-

TABLE 13 *Effects of OK-432, OK-432-stimulated lymphocyte culture supernatant, IFN and IL-2 on generation of auto-tumor killing activity*

Pretreatment of lymphocytes with	% Cytotoxicity to auto-tumor cells	
	Blood lymphocytes	Effusion lymphocytes
Medium	5.3 ± 4.1	5.4 ± 4.8
OK-432	24.9 ± 4.6[a]	21.5 ± 6.4[a]
Supernatant	5.7 ± 2.8	7.1 ± 5.5
IFN	7.0 ± 5.0	7.6 ± 5.7
IL-2	5.0 ± 3.6	7.1 ± 5.0

Blood and effusion lymphocytes were preincubated for 20 h with medium, OK-432 (50 μg/ml), supernatants from 20-h OK-432-stimulated lymphocyte cultures, IFN-α (1,000 U/ml), or IL-2 (33 U/ml), then washed and tested for cytotoxicity against autologous effusion tumor cells at E:T of 40:1. Results are expressed as the mean ±SE of 5 experiments.

a) Value is significantly higher than that of control cells ($p < 0.05$).

tion of OK-432-activated killer cells and resulted in no appearance of cells with blastoid morphology. Furthermore, the three-day culture of lymphocytes with the dose of OK-432 caused complete inhibition of DNA synthesis of lymphocytes even in the presence of mitogens (unpublished data). The possibility that OK-432 stimulates the production of one or more lymphokines in the cytotoxic cells that, in turn, are responsible for the induction of auto-tumor killing activity is currently under investigation.

It has been demonstrated that OK-432 enhances in vivo cytotoxic activity of rat peritoneal macrophages.[4] We therefore conducted experiments to determine whether monocyte/macrophages are involved in the generation of auto-tumor killing activity. Removal of adherent cells on serum-coated plastic dishes and Sephadex G10 columns resulted in no decrease in, and occasionally an increase in, OK-432-induced lysis of autologous tumor cells (Table 14). In addition, blood and effusion adherent cells isolated by adherence to autologous serum-coated plastic dishes were not able to kill autologous fresh effusion tumor cells even after stimulation with OK-432 or IFN. Similarly, the enhancement of NK cell activity by OK-432 was found to be independent of the presence of adherent cells.[10] These results differ from the observations that the generation of cytotoxic cells by lectins requires the presence of adherent cells.[25]

We have demonstrated quite recently that a minor proportion of LGL/NK cells can kill autologous fresh tumor cells in a short-term chromium release assay.[19] It seems of interest and of importance to examine whether the lysis of autologous tumor cells by LGL is augmented by OK-432, or whether other cytotoxic cells are generated by OK-432 to kill autologous tumor cells. As shown in Table 15, LGL isolated by discontinuous Percoll gradient cen-

TABLE 14 *Effects of adherent cells on OK-432-induced lysis of autologous tumor cells*

Effector cells	% Cytotoxicity to auto-tumor	
	Medium	OK-432
Blood		
Unseparated mononuclear cells	1.2 ± 0.6	16.8 ± 9.4[a)]
Lymphocytes	2.6 ± 2.6	23.5 ± 10.2[a)]
Monocytes	0.9 ± 0.6	1.7 ± 1.2
Effusion		
Unseparated mononuclear cells	1.1 ± 1.1	18.5 ± 5.7[a)]
Lymphoid cells	3.1 ± 2.1	24.9 ± 5.3 [a)]
Monocyte/macrophages	0.8 ± 1.0	1.2 ± 1.1

Blood and effusion mononuclear cells were fractionated into lymphocytes and monocyte/macrophages on autologous serum-coated plastic dishes. Each fraction was cultured alone or with OK-432 for 20 h, then washed and tested for cytotoxicity against autologous effusion tumor cells at E:T of 40:1. Results are expressed as the mean ±SE of 3 experiments.
a) Value is significantly higher than that of corresponding control cells ($p < 0.05$).

trifugation expressed significant cytotoxicity against autologous tumor cells, which was enhanced after overnight treatment with OK-432. Both blood and effusion LGL were activated by OK-432 to show enhanced auto-tumor killing activity. In contrast, LGL-depleted T lymphocytes, obtained from high-density fractions of Percoll gradients, were not able to lyse autologous fresh effusion tumor cells even after activation with OK-432. These results indicate that OK-432 augments auto-tumor killing activity of LGL, but not of T lymphocytes. Further studies will be required to determine whether OK-432-induced lysis of autologous fresh tumor cells is exerted by NK cells or by other effector cells. Identification of OK-432-activated killer cells with the use of monoclonal antibodies is in progress.

The next series of experiments were done to ascertain whether xenogeneic serum components are involved in the induction of cytotoxicity against autologous tumor cells. Blood and effusion lymphocytes were cultured for 20 hours, alone or with OK-432, either in human AB serum or FCS, then washed and assayed. Blood and effusion lymphocytes activated with OK-432 in human serum were induced to lyse autologous tumor cells in a four-hour assay (Table 16). No differences were evident in the induction or augmentation of auto-tumor killing activity in human serum and FCS, indicating that xenogeneic serum components are not responsible for the activation of cytotoxic effector cells with OK-432.

TABLE 15 *Effects of OK-432 on auto-tumor killing activity of fractions obtained by discontinuous density gradient centrifugation*

Effector cells	% Cytotoxicity to auto-tumor	
	Medium	OK-432
Blood nonadherent lymphocytes	11.4 ± 2.3	26.8 ± 3.5[a]
Blood LGL	25.8 ± 3.1	45.3 ± 1.9[a]
Blood T lymphocytes	3.3 ± 1.1	6.0 ± 1.7
Effusion nonadherent lymphocytes	18.3 ± 3.0	32.9 ± 6.7[a]
Effusion LGL	30.8 ± 1.8	51.2 ± 5.2[a]
Effusion T lymphocytes	5.1 ± 0.6	8.7 ± 1.9

Blood and effusion nylon-wool nonadherent lymphocytes were fractionated by centrifugation on discontinuous Percoll density gradients. LGL were obtained from fractions 2 and 3 of the gradients and T cells from fractions 6 and 7. Each fraction was incubated alone or with OK-432 for 20 h, then washed and tested for lysis of autologous tumor cells at E:T of 40:1.
a) Value is significantly higher than that of corresponding control cells ($p < 0.05$).

TABLE 16 *Effects of serum on the generation of OK-432-induced lysis of autologous tumor cells*

Effector cells	% Cytotoxicity to auto-tumor			
	FCS with		Human serum with	
	Medium	OK-432	Medium	OK-432
Blood lymphocytes	6.0 ± 2.8	20.8 ± 4.5[a]	5.6 ± 2.7	22.8 ± 5.5[a]
Effusion lymphocytes	5.4 ± 2.9	18.3 ± 3.8[a]	4.1 ± 2.0	18.4 ± 2.3[a]

Blood and effusion lymphocytes were cultured for 20 h, alone or with OK-432, in either FCS or human serum, then washed and tested against autologous effusion tumor cells at E:T of 40:1. Results are expressed as the mean ± SE of 5 experiments.
a) Value is significantly higher than that of untreated lymphocytes ($p < 0.05$).

In vivo induction of auto-tumor killing activity by OK-432

Based on the in vitro findings that OK-432 can cause both peripheral blood and tumor-associated lymphocytes to be cytotoxic against autologous fresh tumor cells, patients with carcinomatous pleural effusions were treated with intrapleural injections of OK-432, since OK-432 therapy has been demonstrated to result in a reduction or complete disappearance of pleural effusions and tumor cells in pleural effusions of cancer patients.[42] Furthermore, we have reported that the reduction or disappearance of effusion tumor cells caused by intrapleural administration of OK-432 is strongly associated with the induction or augmentation of effusion NK cell activity.[7,9] These findings appear to suggest that tumor-associated lymphocytes activated in vivo by OK-432 may interact in vivo with autologous tumor cells in cancer patients. To confirm the above suggestion, patients with carcinomatous pleural effusions were treated with intrapleural injections of OK-432 (10 KE) and monitored for cytotoxicity against autologous effusion tumor cells on day 0 and day 7. Of 12 patients, two (16.7%) had blood and effusion lymphocyte samples which expressed significant lysis of autologous fresh effusion tumor cells on day 0 (Table 17). Seven days after an intrapleural injection of OK-432, no induction of auto-tumor killing activity was observed in the peripheral blood or pleural effusions of non-responder patients who had no clinical benefit from the OK-432 treatment. In contrast, six (85.7%) of seven responder patients, who had a reduction or complete disappearance of tumor cells in their pleural effusions seven days after intrapleural administration of OK-432, had lymphocytes cytotoxic to autologous effusion tumor cells in their pleural effusions on day 7. An induction of auto-tumor killing activity was observed with blood lymphocytes from only one responder patient. It should be noted that an induction or augmentation of auto-tumor killing activity of effusion lymphocytes is associated with the reduction or disappearance of tumor cells in pleural effusions of patients who had received intrapleural administration of OK-432. Furthermore, the induction of effusion auto-tumor killing activity is found to correlate well with an induction or augmentation of effusion NK cell activity. Taken together, our results indicate that OK-432-activated effusion NK cells may effectively kill

TABLE 17 *Induction of auto-tumor killing activity by intrapleural administration of OK-432*

Subjects	Frequency of significant lysis of auto-tumor			
	Blood lymphocytes		Effusion lymphocytes	
	Day 0	Day 7	Day 0	Day 7
Nonresponders (2)[a]	0/2 (0%)	0/2 (0%)	0/2 (0%)	0/2 (0%)
Responders (7)[b]	1/7 (14%)	2/7 (29%)	1/7 (14%)	6/7 (86%)
Responders (3)[c]	1/3 (33%)	1/3 (33%)	—	—

Blood and effusion lymphocytes were tested for cytotoxicity against autologous effusion tumor cells before and 7 days after intrapleural injection of OK-432. Percent cytotoxicity greater than 8% was considered significant.

a) Patients showed no reduction of tumor cells and pleural effusions.
b) Patients showed reduction or disappearance of tumor cells in their effusions.
c) Patients showed complete disappearance of pleural effusions.

autologous tumor cells in vivo in pleural effusions of cancer patients, which could be one mechanism of the reduction or disappearance of tumor cells in pleural effusions of OK-432-treated cancer patients.

Conclusion

It is evident from the data presented in this communication that OK-432 augments NK cell activity of lymphocytes from the peripheral blood, carcinomatous pleural effusions and regional lymph nodes of cancer patients both in vivo and in vitro. In addition, cytotoxic activity against fresh autologous tumor cells was found to be induced or augmented by in vivo and in vitro OK-432 treatment. Although the exact mechanism responsible for the induction or augmentation of natural and auto-tumor killing activities is not understood yet, OK-432 seems to activate cytotoxic cells independently of IFN or IL-2 induction (Table 18). The most practical fact is that OK-432 can induce auto-tumor killing activity of tumor-associated lymphocytes in vivo. It should be noted that OK-432-induced or OK-432-augmented natural killing and auto-tumor killing activities of effusion lymphocytes are strongly associated with the reduction or disappearance of tumor cells in the pleural effusions of cancer patients treated with an intrapleural injection of OK-432. In contrast, there is no correlation between antitumor activity of intrapleural OK-432 therapy and

TABLE 18 *Effects of OK-432, IFN and IL-2 on natural and auto-tumor killing activity*

	OK-432	IFN	IL-2
Augmentation of natural cytotoxicity			
Blood lymphocytes	+++	++	++
Tumor-associated lymphocytes	++	−	±
Lymph node lymphocytes	+	±	+
Blood monocytes	±	+	−
Tumor-associated macrophages	−	−	−
Abrogation of NK suppressor activity			
Tumor-associated macrophages	+++	−	−
Induction of auto-tumor killing activity			
Blood lymphocytes	++	−	−(++)[a]
Tumor-associated lymphocytes	++	−	n.t.
Blood monocytes	−	−	−
Tumor-associated macrophages	−	−	−

+++: Strong effect
++: Moderate effect
+: Weak effect
−: No effect
a) 3–7 days after in vitro treatment.

NK- and auto-tumor killing activities of blood lymphocytes. Taken together, the cytotoxic activity against autologous tumor cells of tumor-associated lymphocytes appears to reflect host resistance against tumors, which could be induced by OK-432 treatment. Thus, immunotherapy with OK-432 will result in a subsequent benefit to cancer patients.

References

1. Aoki, T., Kvedar, J.P., Hollis, V.M. Jr. and Bushar, G.S. (1976): Brief communication: Streptococcus pyogenes preparation OK-432. Immunoprophylactic and immunotherapeutic effects on the incidence of spontaneous leukemia in AKR mice. *J. Natl. Cancer Inst., 56,* 687.
2. Uchida, A. and Hoshino, T. (1980): Clinical studies on cell-mediated immunity in patients with malignant disease. I. Effect of immunotherapy with OK-432 on lymphocyte subpopulation and phytomitogen responsiveness in vitro. *Cancer, 45,* 476.
3. Uchida, A. and Hoshino, T. (1980): Reduction of suppressor cells in cancer patients treated with OK-432 immunotherapy. *Int. J. Cancer, 26,* 401.
4. Ishii, Y., Yamaoka, H., Toh, K. and Kikuchi, K. (1976): Inhibition of tumor growth in vivo and in vitro by macrophages from rats treated with a streptococcal preparation, OK-432. *Gann, 67,* 115.
5. Matsubara, S., Suzuki, F. and Ishida, N. (1979): Induction of immune interferon in mice treated with a bacterial immunopotentiator, OK-432. *Cancer Immunol. Immunother., 6,* 41.
6. Oshimi, K., Kano, S., Takaku, F. and Okumura, K. (1980): Augmentation of mouse natural killer cell activity by a streptococcal preparation, OK-432. *J. Natl. Cancer Inst., 65,* 1265.
7. Uchida, A. and Micksche, M. (1982): Augmentation of NK cell activity in cancer patients by OK-432: Activation of NK cells and reduction of suppressor cells. In: *NK cells and other natural effector cells,* pp. 1303. Editor: R. B. Herberman, Academic Press, New York.
8. Micksche, M., Kokron, O. and Uchida, A. (1982): Clinical and immunopharmacological studies with OK-432, a streptococcal preparation. In: *Current concepts in human immunology and cancer immunomodulation*, pp. 639. Editors: B. Serrou et al., Elsevier Biomedical, Amsterdam and New York.
9. Uchida, A. and Micksche, M. (1983): Intrapleural administration of OK-432 in cancer patients: Activation of NK cells and reduction of suppressor cells. *Int. J. Cancer, 31,* 1.
10. Uchida, A. and Micksche, M. (1981): In vitro augmentation of natural killing activity by OK-432. *Int. J. Immunopharmacol., 3,* 365.
11. Uchida, A. and Micksche, M. (1982): Augmentation of human natural killing activity by OK-432. In: *NK cells and other natural effector cells,* pp.589. Editor: R. B. Herberman, Academic Press, New York.
12. Uchida, A., Micksche, M. and Hoshino, T. (1982): Effect of OK-432 on the natural killer activity of mononuclear cells in circulating blood and carcinomatous pleural effusions. In:*Immunomodulation by microbial products and related synthetic compounds,* pp. 446. Editors: Y. Yamamura et al., Excerpta Medica, Amsterdam.
13. De Vries, J.E., Meyering, M., Van Dongren, A. and Rumke, P. (1975): The influence of different isolation procedures and the use of target cells from melanoma cell lines and short-term cultures on the non-specific cytotoxic effects of lymphocytes

from healthy donors. *Int. J. Cancer, 15,* 391.
14. Becker, S., Kiessling, R., Lee, N. and Klein, G. (1978): Modulation of sensitivity to natural killer cell lysis after in vitro explantation of a mouse lymphoma. *J. Natl. Cancer Inst., 61,* 1495.
15. Zarling, J.M., Eskra, L., Borden, E.C., Horoszewicz, J. and Carter, A. (1979): Activation of human natural killer cells cytotoxic for human leukemia cells by purified interferon. *J. Immunol., 123,* 63.
16. Vose, B.M., Vanky, F. and Klein, E. (1977): Lymphocyte cytotoxicity against autologous tumor biopsy cells in humans. *Int. J. Cancer, 20,* 512.
17. Vose, B.M., Vanky, F., Fopp, M. and Klein, E. (1978): Restricted autologous lymphocytotoxicity in lung neoplasia. Br. *J. Cancer, 38,* 375.
18. Vanky, F., Vose, B.M., Fopp, M. and Klein, E. (1979): Human tumor-lymphocyte interaction in vitro. VI. Specificity of primary and secondary autologous lymphocyte-mediated cytotoxicity. *J. Natl. Cancer Inst., 62,* 1407.
19. Uchida, A. and Micksche, M. (1983): Lysis of fresh human tumor cells by autologous large granular lymphocytes from peripheral blood and pleural effusions. *Int. J. Cancer,* 32, 37.
20. Uchida, A. and Micksche, M. (1983): Lysis of fresh human tumor cells by autologous peripheral blood lymphocytes and pleural effusion lymphocytes activated by OK-432. *J. Natl. Cancer Inst., 71,* 673.
21. Vanky, F., Argov, S.A., Einhorn, S.A. and Klein, E. (1980): Role of alloantigens in natural killing. Allogeneic but not autologous tumor biopsy cells are sensitive for interferon-induced cytotoxicity of human blood lymphocytes. *J. Exp. Med., 151,* 1151.
22. Klein, E. and Vanky, F. (1981): A review. Natural and activated cytotoxic lymphocytes which act on autologous and allogeneic tumor cells. *Cancer Immunol. Immunother., 11,* 183.
23. Allavena, P., Introna, M., Sessa, C., Mangioni, C. and Mantovani, A. (1982): Interferon effect on cytotoxicity of peripheral blood and tumor-associated lymphocytes against human ovarian carcinoma cells. *J. Natl. Cancer Inst., 68,* 555.
24. Strausser, J.L., Mazumder, A., Grimm, E.A., Lotze, M.T. and Rosenberg, S. A. (1981): Lysis of solid tumors by autologous cells sensitized in vitro to alloantigens. *J. Immunol., 127,* 266.
25. Mazumder, A., Grimm, E.A., Zhang, H.Z. and Rosenberg, S.A. (1982): Lysis of fresh human solid tumors by autologous lymphocytes activated in vitro with lectins. *Cancer Res., 42,* 913.
26. Lotze, M.T., Grimm, E.A., Mazumder, A., Strausser, J.L. and Rosenberg, S. A. (1981): Lysis of fresh and cultured autologous tumor by human lymphocytes cultured in T-cell growth factor. *Cancer Res., 41,* 4420.
27. Grimm, E.A., Mazunder, A., Zhang, H.Z. and Rosenberg, S.A. (1982): Lymphokine-activated killer cell phenomenon. Lysis of natural killer-resistant fresh solid tumor cells by interleukin 2-activated autologous human peripheral blood lymphocytes. *J. Exp. Med., 155,* 1823.
28. Timonen, T., Ortaldo, J.R. and Herberman, R.B. (1981): Characteristics of human large granular lymphocytes and relationship to natural killer and K cells. *J. Exp. Med., 153,* 569.
29. Timonen, T., Ortaldo, J.R. and Herberman, R.B. (1982): Analysis by a single cell cytotoxicity assay of natural killer (NK) cell frequencies among human large granular lymphocytes and of the effects of interferon on their activity. *J. Immunol., 128,* 2514.
30. Wakasugi, H., Kasahara, T., Minato, N., Hamuro, H., Miyata, M. and Morioka,

Y. (1982): In vitro potentiation of human natural killer cell activity by a streptococcal preparation, OK-432: interferon and interleukin 2 participation in the stimulation with OK-432. *J. Natl. Cancer Inst., 69,* 807.

31. Herberman, R.B. (Ed.) (1982): NK cells and other natural effector cells. Academic Press, New York.
32. Grimm, E.A. and Bonavida, B. (1979): Mechanism of cell-mediated cytotoxicity at the single cell level. I. Estimation of cytotoxic T lymphocytes frequency and relative lytic efficacy. *J. Immunol., 123,* 2861.
33. Fischer, D.G., Golightly, M.G. and Koren, H.S. (1983): Potentiation of the cytolytic activity of peripheral blood monocytes by lymphokines and interferon. *J. Immunol., 130,* 1220.
34. Moore, M. and Vose, B.M. (1981): Extravascular natural cytotoxicity in man: Anti-K562 activity of lymph node and tumor-infiltrating lymphocytes. *Int. J. Cancer, 27,* 265.
35. Mantovani, A., Allavena, P., Sessa, C., Bolis, G. and Mangioni, C. (1980): Natural killer activity of lymphoid cells isolated from human ascitic ovarian tumors. *Int. J. Cancer, 25,* 573.
36. Uchida, A. and Micksche, M. (1981): Natural killer cells in carcinomatous pleural effusions. *Cancer Immunol. Immunother., 11,* 131.
37. Uchida, A. and Micksche, M. (1981): Suppressor cells for natural killer activity in carcinomatous pleural effusions of cancer patients. *Cancer Immunol. Immunother., 11,* 255.
38. Uchida, A. and Micksche, M. (1982): Suppression of NK cell activity by adherent cells from malignant pleural effusions of cancer patients. In: *NK cells and other natural effector cells,* pp. 1303. Editor: R. B. Herberman, Academic Press, New York.
39. Colotta, F., Rambaldi, A., Introna, M., Colombo, N. and Mantovani, A. (1983): Effect of a streptococcal preparation on natural cytotoxicity in human ovarian carcinoma. *Br. J. Cancer,* (in press).
40. Brunda, M.J., Taramelli, D., Holden, H.T. and Varesio, L. (1983): Suppression of in vitro maintenance and interferon-mediated augmentation of natural killer cell activity by adherent peritoneal cells from normal mice. *J. Immunol., 130,* 1974.
41. Cummingham-Rundles, S. (1982): Control of natural cytotoxicity in the regional lymph node in breast cancer. In: *NK cells and other natural effector cells,* pp. 1133. Editor: R. B. Herberman, Academic Press, New York.
42. Nagao, K., Takizawa, H., Sugita, T. and Watanabe, S. (1979): Treatment of malignant pleural effusion with OK-432, with reference to intercostal tube drainage method. *Cancer Chemother. (Jap.), 6,* 1161.
43. Oshimi, K., Wakasugi, H. Kano, S. and Takaku, F. (1980): Streptococcal preparation OK-432 augments cytotoxic activity against an erythroleukemic cell line in human. *Cancer Immunol. Immunother., 9,* 187.

In vitro effects of OK-432 (picibanil) on immune response in immunodepressed cancer patients

DIDIER CUPISSOL[1], BERNARD SERROU[1] and JEAN P. BUREAU[2]

[1]*Service de Chimio-Immunothérapie et Laboratoire d'Immunopharmacologie des Tumeurs, Montpellier, Cédex and*
[2]*Laboratoire d'Histologie et Immunogénétique, Faculté de Médecine, Nimes, France*

Introduction

For several years immunological investigation of the host-tumor relationship has been carried out on an experimental as well as clinical plane.

We have concentrated attention on two types of cells: first, lymphocytes which form autologous rosettes, and second, natural killer (NK) cells. We have shown that peripheral blood contains a T lymphocyte subpopulation (26%) which is capable of forming autologous rosettes in the presence of red cells and serum from the same donor.[1-2] This subpopulation expresses Fc receptors for IgM, binds OKT4 monoclonal antibodies, expresses neither phenotypic nor functional characteristics of suppressor cells, presents no antibody-dependent cell-mediated cytotoxicity nor NK activity, responds normally to phytohemagglutinin but only weakly to Con A, and is partly responsible for the allogenic and autologous mixed-culture responses. Cancer patients show a sharp and early decrease in these cells just prior to relapse. We have isolated this subpopulation and are presently trying to raise a monoclonal antibody which would more easily characterize these cells. The role of these lymphocytes in the recognition of self and the host-tumor relationship is still not clear. Nevertheless, it has already been shown that this subpopulation is involved in recognition of self, the anti-tumor response, and is sensitive to certain drugs such as the thymic factors.[4]

As for NK activity, we have shown, as other authors before us, that this subpopulation is composed of immature T lymphocytes, most of which carry Fc receptors for IgG. This subpopulation is relatively stable in the cancer patient, except for only the most advanced stages. These cells are radiosensitive and, based on recuperation of this property, serve as a parameter for short term prognosis.

Experimental models

General model and choice of patients: In vitro, we studied the effects of OK-432[3] on isolated peripheral blood lymphocytes from 15 normal donors and 15 solid tumor patients. In vivo testing was evaluated in immune deficient, advanced solid tumor patients (patient selection was based on the guidelines established by the Cancer Immunology and Immunotherapy Group [CI2G]). In two sets of experiments we tested 15 patients: seven breast cancers, five malignant melanomas, and three lung cancers. Patient repartition was seven men and eight women and the mean age was 59 years.

Isolation of lymphocytes: Peripheral blood was obtained from healthy donors and cancer patients who had given their informed consent. The lymphocytes were separated using the Böyum method and washed and adjusted to 1 x 10^6/ml in RPMI medium (Eurobio). Trypan blue dye-exclusion viability was always greater than 95%.

Autorosette-forming cell assay: The method of Caraux et al. was used.[1-2] To obtain autologous rosette formation, lymphocytes were harvested by the Ficoll-metrizoate method, and 0.05 ml of autologous serum was incubated with 0.2 ml of lymphocyte suspension (10^7 cells/ml) for 30 minutes at 4°C. Autologous rosette-forming cells were then added (0.05 ml of a suspension of 3 x 10^8 erythrocytes/ml), and the mixture was centrifuged at 200 g for five minutes and further incubated at 4°C overnight. The tubes were then kept refrigerated, and pellets were resuspended gently by hand. Then 1 ml of Hank's buffered salt solution and 0.1 ml of 0.01% acridine orange were added, and the tubes were kept on ice for at least 30 seconds. The number of cells binding three or more erythrocytes was then scored in a refrigerated hemocytometer under a microscope equipped for fluorescence. This method was thus carried out in an entirely autologous situation, avoiding any allogeneic or xenogeneic interference due to the use of AB serum of fetal calf serum.

Evaluation of NK cell activity: NK cell activity was measured by a ^{51}Cr assay. K562 target cells were labeled with ^{51}Cr and placed in the wells of a Limbro round-bottomed microtest plate with different concentrations of human lymphocytes that had been separated from peripheral blood by the Böyum technique using Ficoll-Metrizoate at 1.077 g/cm^3. The cells were incubated for four hours at 37°C in a humid CO_2 incubator. The statistical analyses were performed using the two-sample t test.[5]

TABLE 1 *Immunopharmacological effects of OK-432 in vitro study*

	1 Healthy donors	2 Cancer patients
Autorosette forming cell assay[a]	12.3 ± 2.8	19.4 ± 3.1
NK activity[b]	41 ± 2.5	48 ± 3.7

a) Lymphocytes were incubated with OK-432 0.5 KE/ml.
b) Lymphocytes were incubated with target cell ratio 25:1 vs 2: $p < 0.05$.

Results

Autorosette-forming cell assay: We observed a significant increase in the number of autologous rosette-forming cells when 10^6 lymphocytes were incubated (Table 1).

NK activity: There was also an increase in NK cell activity when 10^6 lymphocytes were incubated with 0.5 KE/ml of OK-432.

Discussion

In our in vitro study, OK-432 seemed to show an immune response: an increase in autologous responding cells and NK activity. In fact, this work in vitro did not presume the in vivo effects of this drug on the immune system. Recently some authors[6,7] have also demonstrated the increase in NK activity in cancer patients. This increase could be explained by the participation of interferon and interleukin-2 in the stimulation of human natural killer cell activity by OK-432.[8] It seems that the in vitro test in the case of OK-432 could be predictive of the in vivo effects. These results are encouraging and justify an interest for further investigation in order to establish optimal doses and administration schedules as well as to evaluate any placebo effects. The results support a role for OK-432 in association with chemotherapy in the treatment of immunodepressed patients.

References

1. Caraux, J., Thierry, C. and Serrou, B. (1979): Human autologous rosettes: II. Pronostic significance of variations in autologous rosette-forming cells in the peripheral blood of cancer patients. *J. Natl. Cancer Inst., 69,* 593.
2. Caraux, J., Thierry, C., and Esteve, C. Flores, G., Lodise, R. and Serrou, B. (1978): Human autologous rosettes. I. Mechanism of binding of autologous erythrocytes by T cells. *Cell. Immunol., 45,* 36.

3. Moriyasu, F., Miwa, H., and Orika, K. (1980): Immunochemotherapy of gastric cancer with OK-432. In: *Immunomodulation by microbial products and related synthetic compounds*, pp. 442. Editors: Y. Yamamura, S. Kotani, L. Azuma, A. Koda and T. Shisa. Excerpta Medica, Amsterdam.
4. Rucheton, M., Rey, A., Caraux, J., Thierry, C., Esteve, C., Valles, H., Dufer, J., Desplaces, A., Zagury, D. and Serrou, B. (1981): Human autologous rosettes. III. Further characterization: markers and functions. *Cell. Immunol., 64,* 312.
5. Serrou, B. and Dubois, J.B. (1976): Monolayer cell cultures as target cells for the study of lymphocyte cytotoxicity in cancer patients. *Acta Cytol., 20,* 577.
6. Uchida, A., Micksche, M. and Hoshino, T. (1980): Effects of OK-432 on the natural killer activity of mononuclear cells in circulating blood and carcinomatous pleural effusion. In: *Immunomodulation by microbial and related synthetic compounds*, pp. 446. Editors: Y. Yamamura, S. Kotani, L. Azuma, A. Koda and T. Shisa. Excerpta Medica, Amsterdam.
7. Uchida, A. and Micksche, M. (1982): Intrapleural administration of OK-432: In: *Augmentation of natural killer (NK) activity and reduction of NK suppressor pharmacology*, 4, p. 34. Editors: P.W. Muller and J.W. Hadden. Pergamon Press, New York.
8. Wakasugi, H., Kasahara, T., Mirato, N., Hamuro, J. and Miyaka, Y. (1982): In vitro potentiation of human natural killer interferon and interleukin-2 participation with OK-432. *J. Natl. Cancer Inst., 69,* 807.

Successful immunotherapy of carcinomatous pleuritis and peritonitis by intracavitary injection of OK-432

MOTOMICHI TORISU[1], TAKASHI FUJIMURA[1], MASATO KATO[1], MITSUO KATANO[2]*, HIROSHI YAMAMOTO[2]*, KOHKI KONOMI[1], TADANORI MIYATA[1], MASATOSHI KATO[1], TAKESHI YOSHIDA[3]* and MASAKI SAKATA[1]

[1] *The First Department of Surgery, Kyushu University School of Medicine, Fukuoka, Japan*

Introduction

Recently, patients with neoplastic diseases in general, started to enjoy better prognosis than decades ago. However, most advanced cancer patients still have poor prognosis despite the availability of various therapies including immunochemotherapy, irradiation and hormonal therapy. These patients tend to develop effusion in pleural or peritoneal cavities because of obstruction in the lymphatics or the portal vein, hepatic dysfunction, serosal implantation of tumor cells or other causes. The treatment of malignant pleuro-peritoneal effusion has largely been unsatisfactory even when various immuno-chemotherapeutic agents have been used.[1-3] Drainage of the effusion has been the only choice to relieve the symptoms but it usually led to excessive protein and electrolytes loss.

A streptococcal preparation, OK-432, became available,[4-7] and has been in clinical use as an immunomodulator in Japan.[8-10] We have found that patients with malignant effusion who received this agent in the pleural or peritoneal cavity showed not only complete disappearance of effusion but also a significant prolongation of survival time. We have previously reported some such clinical trials and the role of the host's inflammatory cells in tumor cell destruction in ascitic fluid.[11-14] In this communication, we will describe the whole aspect of our study and show the mechanisms of the host's inflammatory cell-mediated tumor cell destruction in malignant effusion.

---

*Present address: [2]Department of Surgery, Saga Medical School, Saga 840-01 Japan
[3]Department of Pathology, The University of Connecticut Health Center, Framington, Connecticut 06032 U.S.A.

The administration of OK-432

OK-432 (Chugai Pharmaceutical Co., Ltd., Tokyo) is produced by incubating the culture of the low virulent Su strain of *Streptococcus pyogenes* of human origin in Bernheimer's basal medium with the addition of penicillin G potassium and then lyophilizing the incubation mixture.[4-6] We used KE (Klinische Einheit) units to express the strength of the preparation. One KE of OK-432 is equivalent to approximately 0. 1 mg of the lyophilized preparation. Intracavitary administration of OK-432 (suspended in 20 ml saline for one to eight weeks until the fluid disappeared)[11] was given weekly at a dosage ranging from 5 to 20 KE.

Patients

A total of two hundred and thirty-two patients with malignant pleuro-peritoneal effusion were treated with either intrapleural or intraperitoneal injections of OK-432 (Table 1). Of these, 129 were males and 103 were females. The mean age of the patients was 58. 4 (range 23-82). The primary lesions with malignancy were as follows: stomach, 136; colon and rectum, 51; breast, 14; biliary tract and pancreas, 10; and others, 21. At the time of this study, none of the patients had been receiving chemotherapeutic agents. Paracentesis was performed when necessary for the patient's comfort.

TABLE 1 *Characteristics of patients with malignant pleuro-peritoneal effusion and therapeutic schedule*

	OK-432 therapy
No. of patients	232
Male: Female	129: 103
Age (mean)	23–82 (58.4)
Gastric cancer	136
Colorectal cancer	51
Breast cancer	14
Biliary tract and pancreas	10
Others	21
Perfomance status	
Grade I	0
Grade II	0
Grade III	44
Grade IV	188
Therapeutic schedule	Intraperitoneal injection of OK-432 Paracentesis, Diuretics, Blood transfusion

Effect of OK-432 therapy on disappearance of effusion

Of the 182 malignant ascites patients treated with OK-432, 112 patients (61.5%) showed complete disappearance or a definite reduction of effusion volume. Both were classified as responders. Thirty-eight of 50 patients with pleural effusion (76%) were responders (Fig. 1). The mean duration from the first administration of OK-432 to disappearance of ascitic fluid and pleural effusion was 22.5 days (range 6-56) and 15.4 (range 1.5-42), respectively (Table 2). However, 70 patients with ascites and 12 with pleural effusion showed no significant change or even an increase in the volume of effusion, despite therapy.

TABLE 2 *Duration from OK-432 injection to disappearance of pleural effusion and ascites*

	No. of patients	Duration: days (mean ± SD)
With ascites	100	6–56 (22.5 ± 7.8)
With pleural effusion	38	1.5–42 (15.4 ± 15.1)

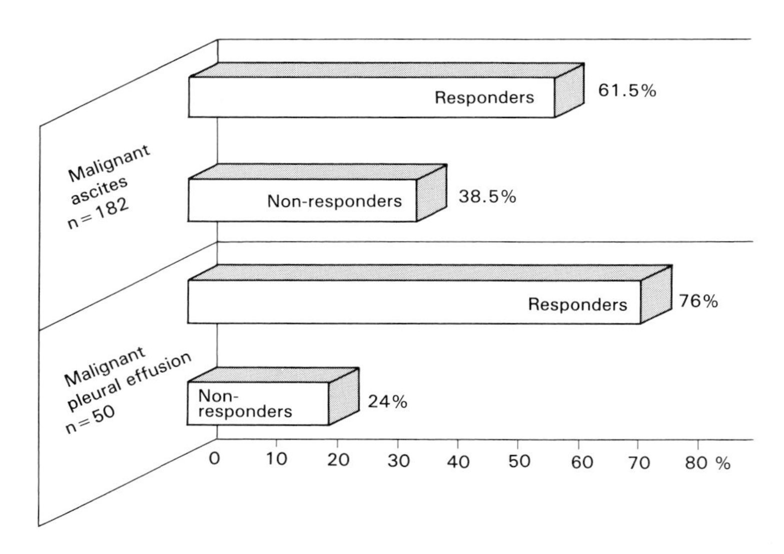

FIGURE 1 *Effect of intraperitoneal or intrapleural injection of OK-432 on disappearance of ascitic fluid and pleural effusion.*
"Responders" represents patients who show complete disappearance or definite reduction of effusion volume. "Non-responders" represents patients who show no significant change or an increase in effusion volume.

Relationship between disappearance of ascites and cytologic findings of ascitic fluid

Cytologic examinations were performed on the ascitic fluid from 150 patients before therapy.[13] Tumor cells were definitely detected in samples from 85 patients and were negative in 65 cases. Interestingly, 68 of 85 patients (80%) with tumor cell positive effusion showed complete disappearance or significant reduction of effusion volume. In contrast, improvement was seen in only 16 of 65 patients (24.6%) with undetectable tumor cells in ascitic fluid (Fig. 2). These results strongly suggest that this therapy is more effective for patients with tumor cell bearing ascites than for those who only have ascitic fluid.

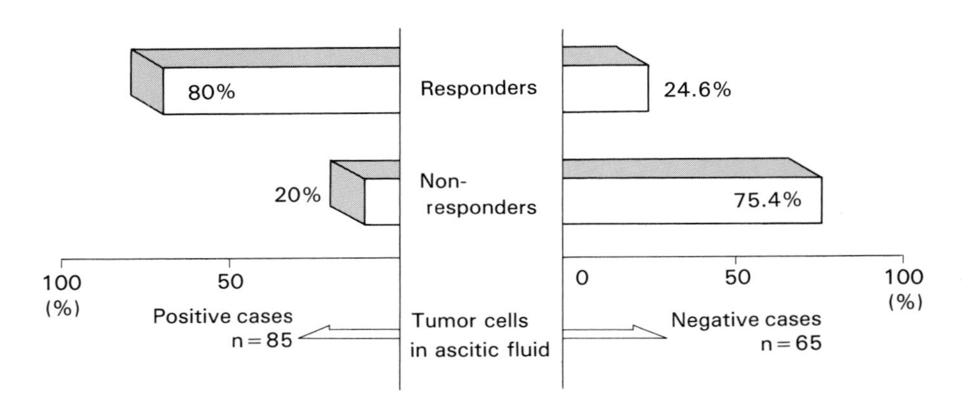

FIGURE 2 *Relationship between disappearance of ascites and cytologic findings of ascitic fluid before the treatment with OK-432.*

Changes in immunologic potency of patients with malignant effusion after the OK-432 therapy

To assess the immunologic capability of patients with malignant effusion, immune responses of patients at stage IV with effusion were compared to those without effusion (Table 3). Methodological details are described elsewhere.[14] All of these parameters were significantly suppressed in patients at stage IV without effusion. In particular, stage IV patients with effusion were remarkably suppressed in all of these parameters. From our experience, usually the immune responses of stage IV patients with effusion show no improvement, even with innoculation of living BCG, which is one of the most powerful immunopotentiators.[15,16] Therefore, the patients with malignant effusion are thought to be in an immunologically deficient state.

Nevertheless, various immunologic parameters usually improved significantly one month after the injection of OK-432.[12] In addition, serum protein

TABLE 3 *Immune responses in patients with malignant pleural effusion and/or ascites*

Immunological parameters	Stage IV (with pleural effusion and/or ascites)	Stage IV (without pleural effusion and ascites)	Healthy volunteers
	200 cases	200 cases	200 cases
Skin tests (% positive)			
PPD	13.8	21.6	91.7
PHA-P	21.4	33.9	97.5
DNCB	16.9	26.4	89.3
KLH	17.1	29.1	95.8
Cellular parameters			
T cell (%)	41.4 ± 20.5	52.5 ± 12.5	65.5 ± 9.9
B cell (%)	49.3 ± 16.3	45.7 ± 8.9	37.4 ± 10.5
Active T cell (%)	2.05 ± 13.4	22.4 ± 12.1	39.0 ± 7.8
Random migration	0.96 ± 0.71	1.99 ± 1.44	4.01 ± 1.15
Chemotactic activity (%)	29.5 ± 17.3	39.9 ± 15.5	101.8 ± 24.1

levels of responders elevated gradually after the therapy. The elevation of serum protein level was closely associated with the decrease in the protein level in ascitic fluid. Therefore, immunologic improvement could be noted after the effusion was reduced. On the other hand, non-responders had no significant change despite the therapy. In the patients who received palliative therapy such as paracentesis, none of these parameters changed.

Survival time

As a result of intracavitary injection of OK-432, the mean survival time of the treated patients was 10.6 months (range 0.2-46) and that of the palliative therapy group was 2.9 months (range 0.2-10.3). This difference was statistically significant ($p<0.05$). When responders (112 cases) were analyzed separately, the mean survival time was 15.6 months (range 2.9-46, $p<0.001$) (Fig. 3). These results indicate that OK-432 therapy induces significant prolongation of the survival time for patients with malignant effusion.

Side effects

This therapy caused some side effects, such as high fever, chill, nausea, abdominal pain and distension (Table 4). High fever was experienced in 149 cases (64.2%) of the OK-432 therapy group. However, it was easily

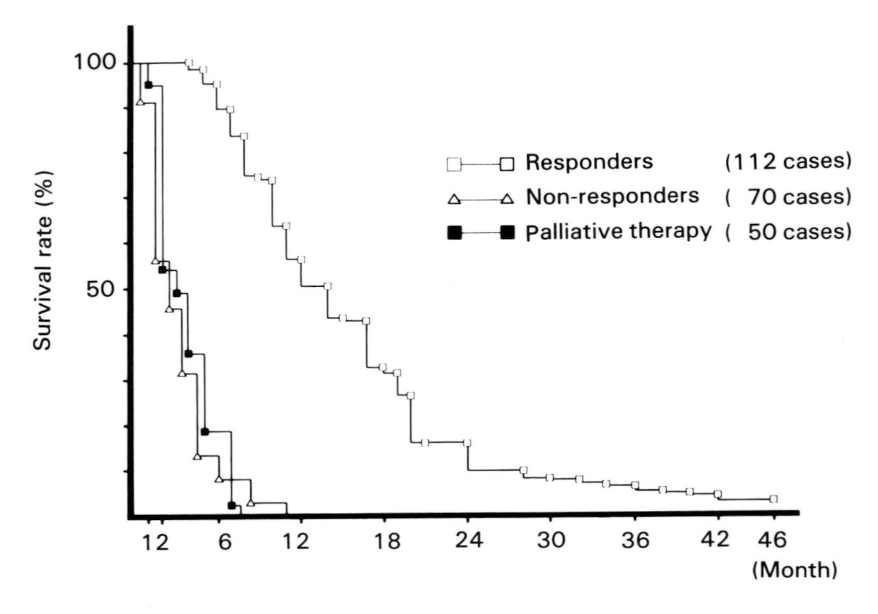

FIGURE 3 *Comparison of survival rate between responders and non-responders or palliative therapy group (Revision of Figure 5 in reference 13).*

TABLE 4 *Side effects of OK-432 therapy in 232 patients*

Clinical signs	No. of patients	Percent (%)
Fever	149	64.2
Chill	71	30.6
Nausea	48	20.6
Headache	8	3.4
Dyspnea	7	3.1
Vomiting	10	4.3
Abdominal pain	43	18.5
Abdominal distension	44	18.9

controlled by anti-febrile medications. Moreover, other serious complications including anaphylactic shock, hepatic dysfunction, renal failure and ileus were not experienced throughout this therapy.

Tumor cell destruction by inflammatory cells

Various inflammatory cells such as neutrophils, macrophages and lymphocytes accumulated in the peritoneal cavity after the injection of OK-432. When

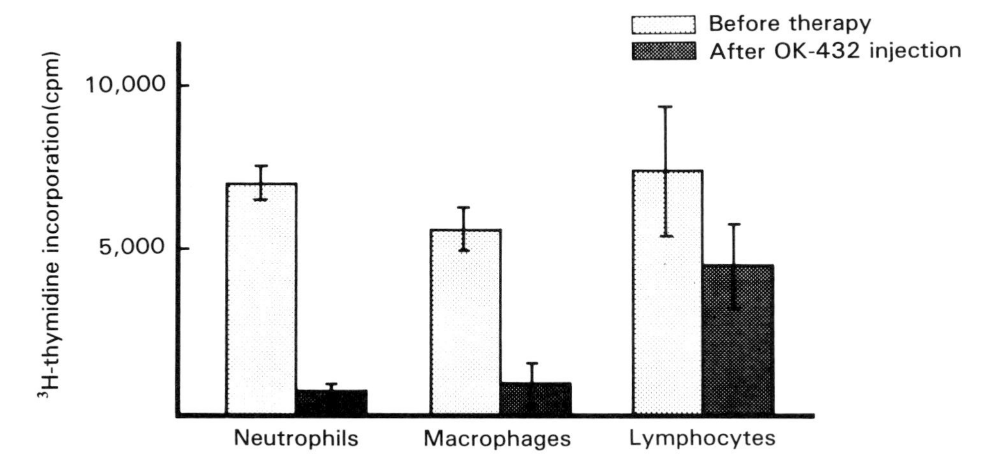

FIGURE 4 *Effect of various inflammatory cells derived from ascitic fluid on DNA synthesis of patient's own tumor cells.*
Rates of effector to target were 100:1 for neutrophils, 10:1 for macrophages and 20:1 for lymphocytes.

smears of ascitic fluid were examined periodically, the inflammatory cells induced by OK-432 adhered to tumor cells and finally destroyed them in vivo.[13] Next, the effect of inflammatory cells from ascitic fluid after the treatment with OK-432 on DNA synthesis of the patient's own tumor cells was studied by in vitro tritium-thymidine incorporation.[11,12] DNA synthesis of tumor cells was significantly inhibited by the activated inflammatory cells (Fig. 4). These results suggest that the host's inflammatory cells play an important role in tumor cell destruction in malignant effusion.

Role of neutrophils in tumor cell destruction

Various agents such as OK-432, BCG, mitomycin C and adriamycin were previously given intrapleurally or intraperitoneally for patients with malignant effusion. When the ascitic fluid was cytologically examined after the administration of these agents, a predominant accumulation of neutrophils was the characteristic feature for OK-432 (Table 5).

Figure 5 represents a typical case who showed characteristic changes in the number of neutrophils and tumor cells in the peritoneal cavity. There were many tumor cells and only a few neutrophils in the effusion before the treatment with OK-432. Following the treatment, neutrophils strikingly increased in number within 24 hours. Infiltrating neutrophils gradually decreased on the second day. In contrast, tumor cells clearly decreased in number soon after the administration of OK-432 and slightly increased on the 6th day. After an additional injection of OK-432 on the 7th day, the

TABLE 5 *Changes of inflammatory cells appearing in ascitic fluid after intraperitoneal administration of various agents*

Agents	24 hours			96 hours		
	Neutrophil	Lymphocyte	Macrophage	Neutrophil	Lymphocyte	Macrophage
OK-432	++++	±	±	++	+++	+++
BCG	+	++	±	+	+++	+
Mitomycin C	−	±	−	−	±	−
Adriamycin	−	−	−	−	−	−
Palliative therapy	−	−	−	−	−	−

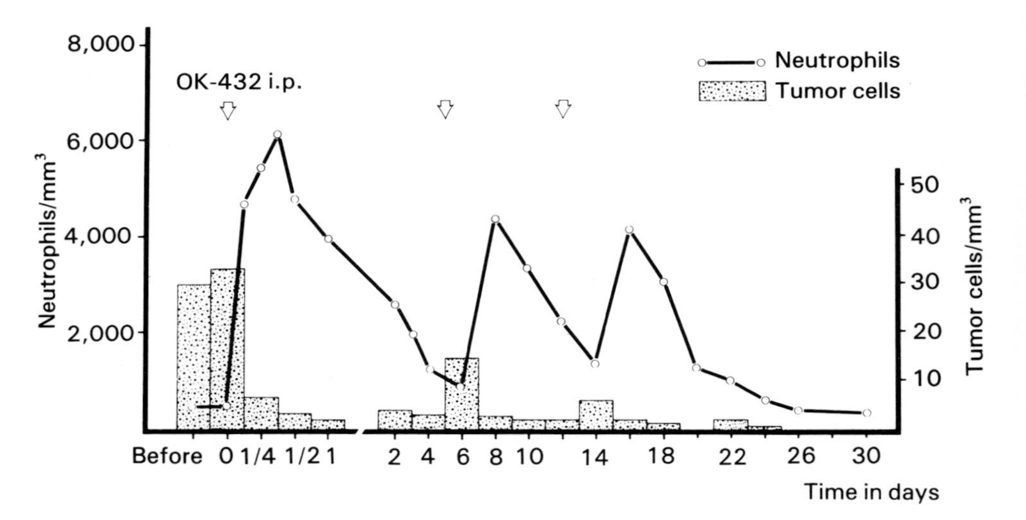

FIGURE 5 *Typical change in numbers of intraperitoneal neutrophils and tumor cells after OK-432 injection.*

numbers of neutrophils and tumor cells showed a similar pattern to that after the first injection. Usually, tumor cells disappeared completely after several injections of OK-432.

In order to clarify the mechanisms of neutrophil accumulation, neutrophil chemotactic activity of ascitic fluid was measured in vitro by Boyden's chamber technique.[18] Interestingly, the chemotactic activity of ascitic fluid increased remarkably after the OK-432 administration.[18] In addition, after an incubation of ascitic fluid with OK-432 in vitro, the chemotactic activity significantly increased in comparison with that of OK-432-free ascitic fluid. However, OK-432 itself was repeatedly shown not to have the chemotactic activity for neutrophils. From these results, it is apparent that a chemoattractant for neutrophils is generated as a consequence of the ascitic fluid and OK-432 interaction.

We examined the morphological process of tumor cell destruction by an ascitic fluid smear on glass slides (Fig. 6). After the injection, neutrophils induced by OK-432 surrounded clusters of tumor cells, adhered tightly to them and infiltrated into the tumor clusters. The clusters finally dispersed to a number of single tumor cells by such neutrophils. Some neutrophils invaded the cytoplasm of tumor cells and destroyed them. These observations indicate that neutrophils induced by OK-432 may play the most important role in tumor cell disappearance from ascitic fluid.

The possible mechanism for the disappearances of tumor cells and ascitic fluid from the peritoneal cavity

Two different pathways may cause the disappearance of tumor cells in an effusion after the administration of OK-432 (Fig. 7). The first pathway is shown by solid arrows in Figure 7. Thus, the inflammatory cells activated by OK-432 adhere, infiltrate, disperse the cluster of tumor cells and finally destroy tumor cells in the effusion. The second is shown by broken arrows in Figure 7. These activated cells may also attack metastatic sites in peritoneum. Tumor cells may not be able to leave metastatic sites for the peritoneal cavity, because the tumor is covered with fibrotic tissue after the surface of the tumor is damaged by the inflammatory cells. These two pathways may contribute to the disappearance of tumor cells from the peritoneal cavity.

The possible mechanisms of fluid disappearance from peritoneal cavity are shown in Figure 8. Complement system in ascitic fluid activated by OK-432 releases anaphilatoxins and chemotactic factors, which causes inflammation of the peritoneum. The production of fluid is decreased because of the damage of endotherial cells in peritoneum and deposition of fibrotic tissue. In addition, the absorption of fluid may be enhanced due to the elevation of the serum protein level.

In 8 years of experience with OK-432 therapy in cancer patients, we have found that inflammatory cells, especially neutrophils, play an important role in tumor cell destruction in the peritoneal as well as pleural cavity and we believe that OK-432 therapy is the best choice for treatment of malignant pleuro-peritoneal effusion among the various therapies at the present time.

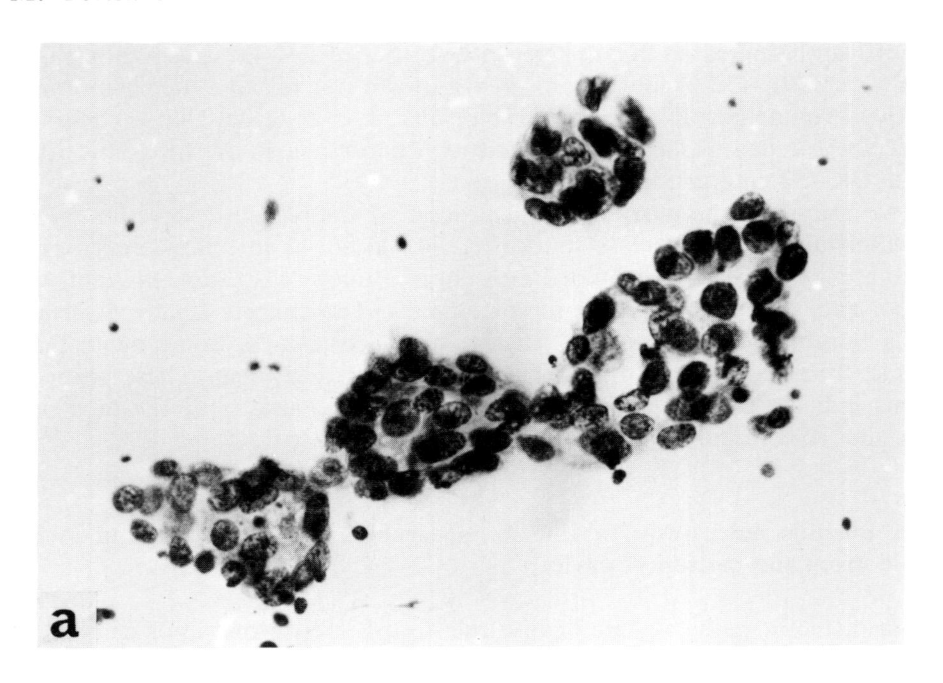

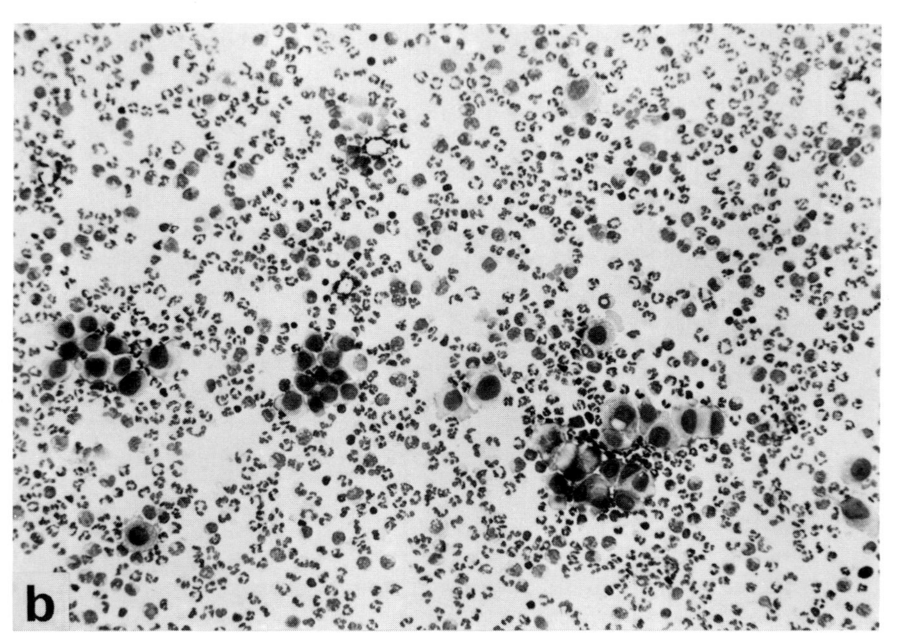

FIGURE 6 *Representative patient showing tumor cell destruction by neutrophils on glass slide.*
a) Clusters of tumor cells without many inflammatory cells.
b) Clusters of tumor cells surrounded by infiltrating neutrophils.

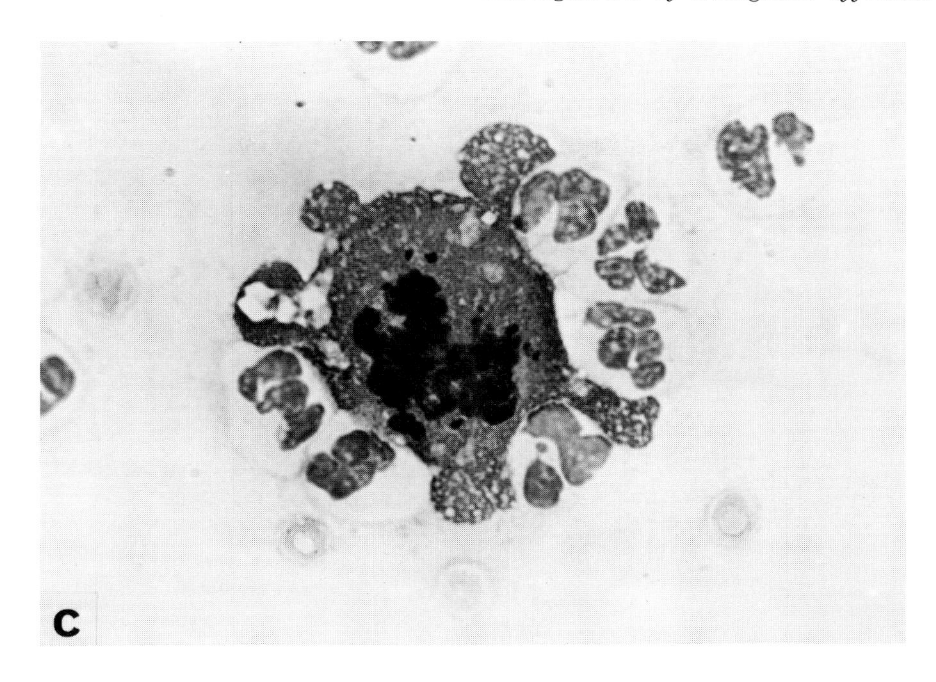

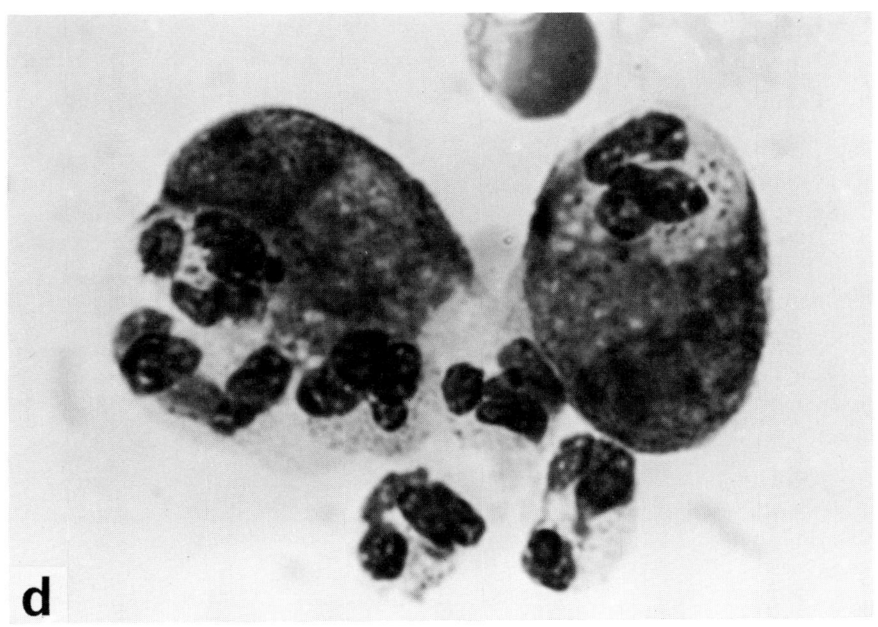

FIGURE 6 *Representative patient showing tumor cell destruction by neutrophils on glass slide.*
c) A tumor cell surrounded by infiltrating neutrophils.
d) A tumor cell cytoplasm invaded by infiltrating neutrophils.

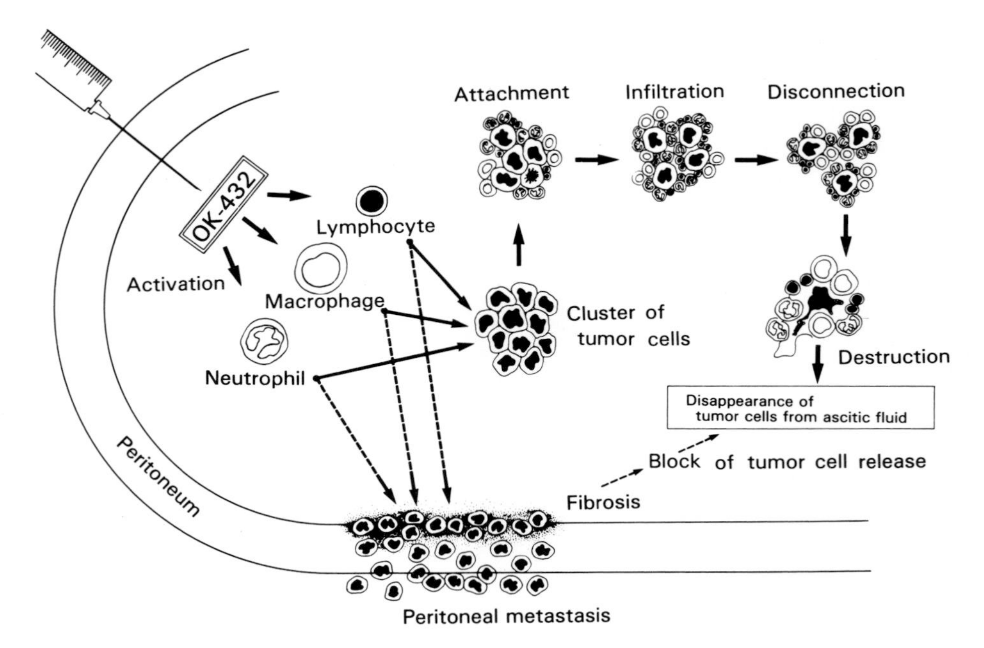

FIGURE 7 *The possible mechanisms of tumor cell disappearance in ascitic fluid.* Solid arrows indicate the first pathway, and the broken arrows the second pathway.

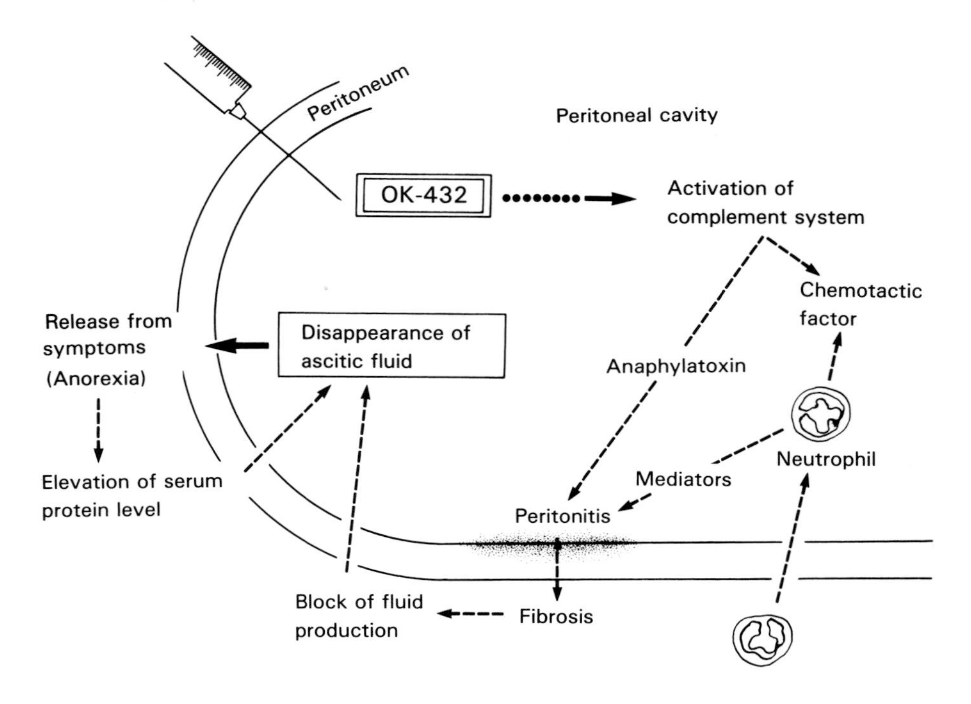

FIGURE 8 *The possible mechanisms of fluid disappearance in peritoneal cavity.*

Summary

Two hundred and thirty-two patients with pleural or peritoneal effusion caused by various types of cancer were treated with either an intrapleural or intraperitoneal injection of a streptococcal preparation, OK-432. Effusion disappeared in 112 of 182 patients with ascites (61.5%) and 38 of 50 patients with pleural effusion (76%). The effect of this therapy appeared to be dependent on the cytologic nature of the effusion prior to treatment. The effusion which initially contained tumor cells, disappeared in 68 of 85 patients (80%). On the other hand, only 16 out of 65 patients (24.6%) with tumor cell-free effusion responded to the therapy. The results indicate that this therapy is more effective in patients with effusion bearing tumor cells ($p<0.001$). The mean survival time of all patients with ascites was 10.6 months (range 0.2-46). When analyzing only the responders (112 case), the mean survival time was 15.6 months, while that of non-responders and palliative therapy groups was 2.7 and 2.9 months, respectively. Thus, the therapy with OK-432 significantly prolonged the survival time ($p<0.001$). During the treatment, various inflammatory cells including neutrophils, macrophages or lymphocytes accumulated in the peritoneal and pleural cavity, and they seemed to attach to tumor cells and finally destroy them. Moreover, such inflammatory cells induced by OK-432 inhibited in vitro DNA synthesis of tumor cells. These results strongly suggest that the host's inflammatory cells induced by OK-432 play an important role in tumor cell destruction in malignant effusion.

References

1. Paladine, W., Cunningham, T.J., Sponzo, R., Donavan, M., Olson, K. and Horton, J. (1976): Intracavitary bleomycin in the management of malignant effusions. *Cancer, 38,* 1903.
2. Suhrland, L.G. and Weisberger, A.S. (1965): Intracavitary 5-fluorouracil in malignant effusions. *Arch. Intern. Med., 116,* 431.
3. Webb, H.E., Oaton, S.W. and Pike, C.P. (1978): Treatment of malignant ascite and pleural effusion with Corynebacterium parvum. *Br. Med. J., l,* 338.
4. Koshimura, S., Shimizu, R., Fujimura, A. and Okamoto, H. (1964): Experimental anticancer studies XXI. Effect of penicillin treatment of hemolytic streptococcus on its anticancer activity. *Gann, 55,* 233.
5. Okamoto, H., Shoin, S., Koshimura, S. and Shimizu, R. (1966): Experimental anticancer studies part XXXI. On the streptococcal preparation having potent anticancer activity. *Jap. J. Exp. Med., 36,* 175.
6. Sakurai, Y., Tsukagoshi, S., Satoh, H., Akiba, T. , Suzuki, S. and Takagaki, Y. (1972): Tumor-inhibitory effect of a streptococcal preparation (NSC-B116209). *Cancer Chemother. Rep., 56,* 9.
7. Sakai, S., Ryoyama, K., Koshimura, S. and Migita, S. (1976): Studies on the properties of a streptococcal preparation OK-432 (NSC-B116209) as an immunopotentiator. I. *Jap. J. Exp. Med., 46,* 123.

8. Kimura, T., Ohnishi, T., Yasuhara, S., Sugiyama, M., Urabe, Y., Fujii, M. and Machida, K. (1976): Immunochemotherapy in human lung cancer using the streptococcal agent OK-432. *Cancer, 37,* 2201.
9. Uchida, A. and Hoshino, T. (1980): Clinical studies on cell-mediated immunity in patients with malignant disease. I. Effect of immunotherapy with OK-432 on lymphocyte subpopulation and phytomitogen responsiveness in vitro. *Cancer, 45,* 476.
10. Watanabe, Y. and Iwa, T. (1982): Results of immunotherapy by streptococcal preparation OK-432 as an adjuvant for resected lung cancer. *Proc. 13th Intern. Cancer Congr.,* Seattle, 358.
11. Katano, M. and Torisu, M. (1982): Neutrophil-mediated tumor cell destruction in cancer ascites. *Cancer, 50,* 62.
12. Torisu, M., Katano, M., Kimura, Y. and Itoh, H. (1983): Approach to management of malignant ascites with a streptococcal preparation, OK-432. I. Improvement of host immunity and prolongation of survival. *Surgery, 93,* 357.
13. Torisu, M., Sakata, M., Fujimura, T., Itoh, H., Kimura, Y., Takesue, M., Yoshida, T. and Katano, M. (1984): Successful treatment of malignant ascites: Clinical evaluation and role of host's inflammatory cells in tumor cell destruction in ascites. In: *Basic Mechanisms and Clinical Treatments of Tumor Metastasis,* Editors: M. Torisu and T. Yoshida. Acad. Press, New York. (in press)
14. Torisu, M., Fukawa, M., Nishimura, M., Harasaki, H., Kai, S. and Tanaka, J. (1976): Immunotherapy of cancer patients with BCG: Summary of four years experience in Japan. In: *International Conference on Immunotherapy of Cancer,* Vol. 277, pp. 160. Editors: C. H. Southman and H. Friedman. Ann. N. Y. Acad. Sci., New York.
15. Morton, D.L., Eilber, F.R., Malmgren, R.A. and Wood, W.C. (1970): Immunological factors which influence response to immunotherapy in malignant melanoma. *Surgery, 68,* 158.
16. Gutterman, J.U., Mavlight, G., McBride, C., Frei, E. III, Freireich, E.J., and Hersh, E.M. (1973): Active immunotherapy with B.C.G. for recurrent malignant melanoma. *Lancet, 1,* 1208.
17. Boyden, S.V. (1951): The absorption of proteins on erythrocytes treated with tannic acid and subsequent hemagglutination by antiprotein sera. *J. Exp. Med., 93,* 107.
18. Fujimura, T., Katano, M., Sakata, M. and Torisu, M. (1983): New clinical management of malignant ascites: The mechanism of neutrophil accumulation in ascitic fluid. *Fred. Proc., 42,* 680.

The effect of OK-432 (picibanil) on immunoparameter studies and survival in patients with stage III stomach cancer

JIN-POK KIM, JAE-GAHB PARK and SANG-JOON KIM

Department of Surgery, College of Medicine, Seoul National University and Seoul National University Hospital, Seoul, Korea

Introduction

Since the 1960s, the importance of postoperative adjuvant therapy has been emphasized and therapy for gastric cancer has been turned towards multimodality therapy combining the surgery, radiotherapy, chemotherapy, and immunotherapy. After the gastric cancer cells are reduced as much as possible by radical surgery, it is the ultimate goal of adjuvant immunochemotherapy to irradicate the remaining cancer cells or micrometastases and to cure the patient. Chemotherapy of gastric cancer evolved gradually from single agent chemotherapy to combination chemotherapy after the Japanese report[1] of the 55% response rate with the combination of mitomycin C, 5-FU, and cytosine arabinoside (MFC) and Mortel's report[2] of the 44% response rate with the combination of 5-FU and methyl-CCNU in patients with advanced gastric cancer. The further the clinical stage of gastric cancer is advanced, the more the cell mediated immunity of host is depressed.[3,4] Therefore, enhancement of depressed immune status of host is also an important step of treatment. The purpose of this study was to know the therapeutic effectiveness of immunochemotherapy after radical subtotal gastrectomy for patients with stage III gastric cancer.

Materials and methods

Patients: During the period between 1975 and 1980, 73 patients with stage III gastric cancer treated with radical subtotal gastrectomy followed by immunochemotherapy at the Department of Surgery, Seoul National University Hospital were included in this study. The control group was 64 patients with stage III gastric cancer treated with radical subtotal gastrectomy alone during the period between 1970 and 1980. None had previously been treated with radiotherapy of chemotherapy. The initial performance status was within the range of ECOG (Eastern Cooperative Oncology Group) 0-2 in all patients.

Patient's survival rate: Post-treatment survival in two groups were calculated by Chin Long Chiang's life table method.

Postoperative immunochemotherapy (Table 1)

a) Immunotherapy: OK-432 (Streptococcal preparation) was administered i.m. weekly with the dosage of 1.0 K.E. (Klinische Einheit) from the 4th or 5th POD.
b) Chemotherapy: MFC regimen or FME regimen was selected at random to the patients and started at the 8th to 10th POD. Drug dosage was modified based upon the parameters of hematologic toxicities and other adverse reactions.

Immunological studies

a) *DNCB skin test*: 0.1 ml of 2% DNCB (1-chloro-2, 4-nitrobenzene) solution (sensitizing dose) and 0.05% DNCB solution (challenge dose) were smeared over a 2 cm area of inner surface of arm. The reaction was evaluated by the scale of ++++, +++, ++, +, and 0.
b) *T lymphocyte percent and count:* Lymphocytes were isolated using the Ficoll-Hypaque method from the heparinized peripheral blood of patients. They were mixed with washed sheep RBC and incubated for 18 hours at 37°C. After incubation, the number of rosette-forming cells with at least 3 sheep RBCs was counted among 200 lymphocytes, and it was represented as the percent of T-cells.
c) *The degree of lymphoblastogenesis by PHA and Concanavalin A stimulation:* Lymphocytes were prepared by the Ficoll-Hypaque method from the peripheral blood of patients. 0.1 ml of PHA and 50 μg of Con A were added to 0.2 ml of cell suspension (1.5×10^6 cells) and 3 ml of TC-199 media, respectively. They were incubated for 72 hours under the presence of 5% CO_2. Four hours prior to harvest, 0.5 μCi of tritiated thymidine was added to each culture tube. Cells were harvested and their radioactivity was determined using a scintillation counter.
d) *ADCC (Antibody Dependent Cellular Cytotoxicity) activity:* Lymphomononuclear cells isolated from the peripheral blood of patients, ^{51}Cr-labelled chicken red blood cells, anti-chicken red blood cell antibody from rabbit, and 10% FCS-RPMI media were mixed together and incubated for 18 hours at 37°C. After culturing, the radioactivity of the supernatant was determined. The ratio of lymphomononuclear cells (effector cell) to ^{51}Cr-labelled chicken RBCs (target cell) was 10 to 1. Cytotoxicity was calculated from the formula;

$$^{51}\text{Cr release } (\%) = \frac{\text{experimental release} - \text{spontaneous release}}{\text{maximum release} - \text{spontaneous release}} \times 100$$

TABLE 1 *Postoperative immunochemotherapy programs evaluated in this study*

Duration: 1 year and 6 months		
Chemotherapy—starts at the 8th-10th POD.		
—Mitomycin C	4 mg/50 kg	I.V. ×2/wk for 2 wks, then weekly 6 times
5-fluorouracil	500 mg/50 kg	
cytosine arabinoside	40 mg/50 kg	
followed by oral 5-FU (Futraful) 600 mg, daily		
—oral 5-FU (Futraful) 400 mg/M^2, daily		
oral methyl CCNU, 150 mg/M^2, every 6 weeks		
Immunotherapy—starts at the 4th-5th POD.		
—OK-432 (*Streptococcus pyogenes* preparation)		
1.0 K.E., i.m., weekly		

Results

Survival: The survival curves for each treatment group is presented in Figure 1. 1-yr, 2-yr, 3-yr, 4-yr, and 5-yr-survival rates in the postoperative immunochemotherapy group were 93%, 74.2%, 55.5%, 49.8% and 38.1%, respectively and those in surgery alone group were 87.2%, 58.7%, 41.6%, 32.4%, and 24.8%, respectively. Superior survival for patients who received postoperative immunochemotherapy compared to that for patients who received surgery alone was demonstrated and this difference of approximately 15% in survival was evident and rather constant with a more than 2-year follow-up ($p<0.01$). Median survival was 28 months in the surgery alone group and 42 months in the postoperative immunochemotherapy group.

DNCB skin test: The preoperative DNCB positivity was 47.4% in the surgery alone group and 54.8% in the postoperative immunochemotherapy group, and DNCB positivity at the postoperative 4th month was 73% in the surgery alone group and 92.9% in the postoperative immunochemotherapy group. More patients were converted from a negative DNCB test to a positive DNCB test after postoperative immunochemotherapy (Figure 2).

T lymphocyte percent and count: T lymphocyte percent and count decreased by $2.4 \pm 10.4\%$ and $157 \pm 603/mm^3$ after surgery in the surgery alone group, but increased by $3.2 \pm 8.1\%$ and $46 \pm 740/mm^3$ after therapy in the postoperative immunochemotherapy group (Figure 2).

Degree of lymphoblastogenesis by PHA and Con A stimulation: Degrees of lymphoblastogenesis by PHA and Con A stimulation were decreased by 1,882.4 ± 872 cpm and 4,243.1 ± 1,196 cpm after surgery in the surgery alone group, but they were much less decreased by 404 ± 789.2 cpm and

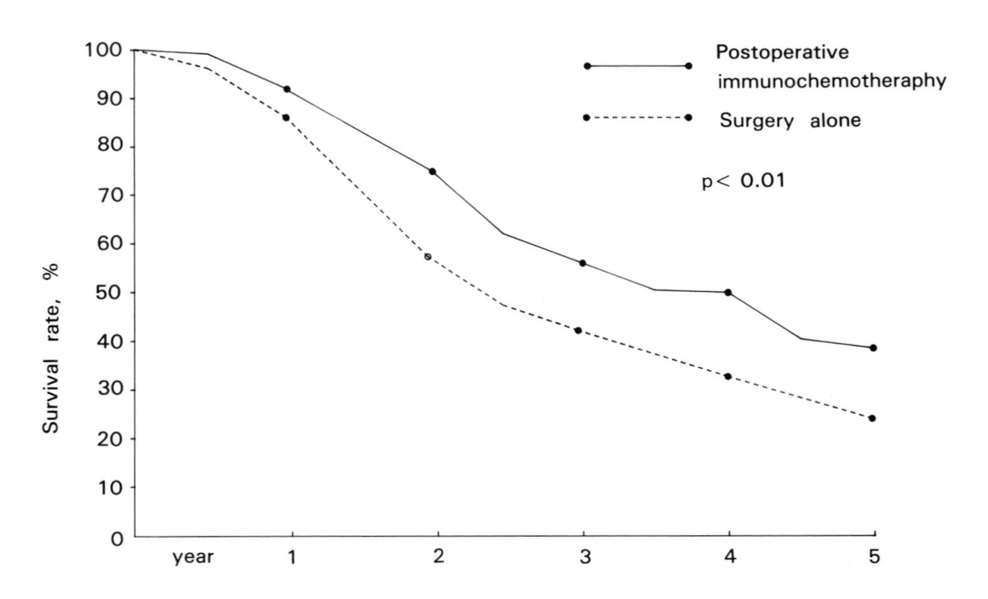

FIGURE 1 *Survival rate of postoperative immunochemotherapy group (n=73) and surgery alone group (n=64).*

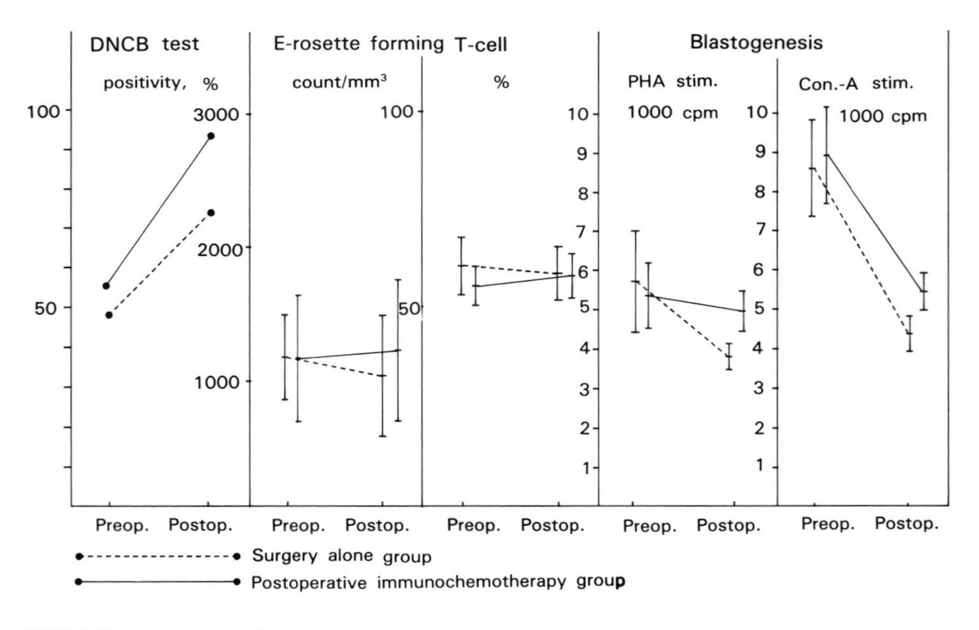

FIGURE 2 *Various immunoparameter studies in stage III gastric cancer patients of surgery alone group and postoperative immunochemotherapy group.*

TABLE 2 *ADCC activity (%) in surgery alone group and postoperative immunochemotherapy group*

	No. of cases	ADCC% ^{51}Cr release	
		Preop. level	Postop. level*
Surgery alone group	28	37.4 ± 12.0	37.9 ± 13.5
Postoperative immuno-chemotherapy group	49	37.7 ± 11.9	39.4 ± 10.3

*ADCC activity at the postoperative 90 day
Note: ADCC activity (%) in 49 normal healthy persons: 44.0 ± 15.9

3,470 ± 1,250.6 cpm after therapy in the postoperative immunochemotherapy group (Figure 2).

Antibody dependent cellular cytotoxicity (ADCC) activity: The preoperative ADCC activity (%) was 37.4 ± 12.0% in the surgery alone group and 37.7 ± 11.9% in the postoperative immunochemotherapy group, and that at the postoperative 3rd month was 37.9 ± 13.5% in the surgery alone group and 39.4 ± 10.3% in the postoperative immunochemotherapy group ($p > 0.1$) (Table 2).

Discussion

Since the 1970s, oncologists have expected that the adjuvant therapy after radical gastric resection for stomach cancer may increase the survival and even cure the patients, but there was no long-term (at least 5 years follow-up) data for that. There are pessimistic reports that the postoperative adjuvant therapy does not increase the survival of patients with gastic cancer.[5-9.] This study shows a much better 5-year survival rate in the postoperative immunochemotherapy group than in the surgery alone group. There are two characteristics in this study; first, we performed the radical subtotal gastrectomy as thoroughly as possible. The regional lymph nodes including the adjacent tissues were removed in *en bloc* fashion using the frozen biopsy.

It is true that stage III gastric cancer is already a systemic disease[10] and can't be cured with local therapy alone, though the loco-regional therapy may be performed thoroughly and aggressively. But the complete removal of tumor cells is of prime importance among the multimodality therapy for cancer and surgery itself is immunotherapy. Secondly, we started the adjuvant immunochemotherapy early after surgery. In general, the adjuvant chemotherapy was performed between 3 and 6 weeks following the operation, but we initiated the immunotherapy at the postoperative 4th or 5th day and the chemotherapy at the postoperative 8th to 10th day. The purpose of this early postoperative adjuvant therapy was to achieve a cure by destroying the tumor cells including the micrometastases when the body burden of tumor cells was the lowest. Gunduz and Fisher[11] provided the important rationale of early postsurgical use of adjuvant chemotherapy. Nissen-Meyer et al.[12] reported a reduction in the recurrence rate and death rate with adjuvant chemotherapy immediately after mastectomy for breast cancer, but not with the same chemotherapy given 3 weeks after mastectomy. We never observed the problem of wound healing with early chemotherapy.

The effectiveness of postoperative immunochemotherapy has been debatable. Makowka[13] reported the ineffectiveness of adjuvant immunochemotherapy with 5-FU and BCG for gastric cancer, but Suga et al.[14] reported the longer survival in patients treated with the immunochemotherapy of MFC and OK-432 compared to patients treated with MFC alone for advanced gastric cancer. We intended to alleviate the immunosuppression caused by chemotherapy with the use of an immunopotentiator. The various immune parameter data in this study showed much better results in the postoperative adjuvant immunochemotherapy group than in the surgery alone group. We continued the postoperative adjuvant immunochemotherapy for 18 months and it seems that better results were obtained when the duration of adjuvant therapy was over 1 year. The postoperative immunochemotherapy is no longer adjuvant therapy, but an important systemic therapeutic means to cure the cancer patient. The authors propose to take out the word "adjuvant" and to call the multimodality therapy of radical surgery, postoperative chemotherapy, and immunotherapy as "Immunochemosurgery". The gastric cancer patient, we believe, can be cured with active immunochemosurgery in the future. To reach that goal, many prospective, controlled clinical studies on immunochemosurgery should be done.

Summary

The effects of immunochemosurgery on 73 patients with stage III gastric cancer treated with radical subtotal gastrectomy followed by immunochemotherapy for 18 months during the period between 1975 and 1980 were compared to the effects of therapy on 64 patients with stage III gastric cancer treated with radical subtotal gastrectomy alone during the period between 1970 and 1980. For immunotherapy, OK-432 (Streptococcal preparation) was intramuscularly given weekly, and for chemotherapy, either MFC (mitomycin C, 5-FU, and cytosine arabinoside) regimen i.v. 10 times followed by oral 5-FU or FME (5-FU and methyl-CCNU) regimen was given. A superior survival for patients who received postoperative immunochemotherapy compared to that for patients who received surgery alone was demonstrated and this difference of approximately 15% in survival was evident and rather constant with a more than 2-year follow-up ($p<0.01$).

Various immune parameter studies such as the DNCB test, T lymphocyte count and percent, PHA and Concanavalin A stimulated lymphoblastogenesis, and ADCC activity showed more favorable data in the postoperative immunochemotherapy group than in the surgery alone group. The radical gastrectomy followed by early postoperative immunochemotherapy (immunotherapy at 4-5 POD and chemotherapy at 8-10 POD) seems to be superior to surgery alone for stage III gastric cancer.

References

1. Kazua, O. et al. (1972): Combination therapy with mitomycin C, 5-fluorouracil and cytosine arabinoside for advanced cancer in man. *Cancer Chemother. Rept., 56*, 373.
2. Moertel, C.G. et al. (1976): Sequential and combination chemotherapy of advanced gastric cancer. *Cancer, 38*, 678.
3. Kim, J.P., and Yoo, I.H. (1978): Relationship between the advance of stomach cancer and the change in immunity. *J. Korean Surg. Soc., 20*, 195.
4. Orita, K. et al. (1976): Preoperative cell-mediated immune status of gastric cancer patient. *Cancer, 38*, 2343.
5. Blake, J.R.S. et al. (1981): Gastric cancer: A controlled trial of adjuvant chemotherapy following gastrectomy. *Clin. Oncol., 7*, 13.
6. Dixon, W.J., Longmire, W.P., Holden, W.D. (1971): Use of triethylenethiophosphoramide as an adjuvant to the surgical treatment of gastric and colorectal carcinoma: Ten year follow-up. *Ann. Surg., 173*, 16.
7. Huguier, M. et al. (1980): Gastric carcinoma treated by chemotherapy after resection. A controlled study. *Am. J. Surg., 139*, 197.
8. Koyama, Y., Kimura, T. (1978): Controlled clinical trials of chemotherapy as an adjuvant to surgery in gastric carcinoma. International Cancer Congress, Buenos Aires, Proc. II, p. 1-21.
9. Serlin, O. et al. (1977): Factors related to survival following resection for gastric carcinoma. Analysis of 903 cases. *Cancer, 40*, 1318.
10. Papachristou, D.N., Fortner, J.G. (1981): Is gastric cancer generalized at the time of surgery? *J. Surg. Oncol., 18*, 27.
11. Gunduz, N., Fisher, B., and Saffer, E.A. (1979): Effect of surgical removal on the growth and kinetics of residual tumor. *Cancer Res., 39*, 3861.
12. Nissen-Meyer, et al., (1978): Surgical adjuvant chemotherapy: Results with one short course with cyclophosphamide after mastectomy for breast cancer. *Cancer, 41*, 2088.
13. Makowka, J. et al. (1980): Adjuvant chemoimmunotherapy for gastric carcinoma. *Can. J. Surg., 23*, 429.
14. Suga, S. et al. (1977): Treatment of gastric cancer with special reference to the survivals of the cancer patients treated with multiple combination MFC therapy or immunochemotherapy of MFC plus OK-432 (NSC B116209). *Gastroenterol. Jpn., 12*, 20.

Clinical value of immunotherapy by streptococcal preparation, OK-432, for lung cancer: A randomized study

YOH WATANABE and TAKASHI IWA

Department of Surgery, Kanazawa University School of Medicine, Kanazawa, Japan

Introduction

There is a decrease of immunity in cancer patients. In lung cancer patients immunological impairment is more conspicuous than in other forms of cancer, and this impairment is exacerbated further by surgical intervention, radiation therapy, or chemotherapy itself.

In 1976 McKneally et al.[1] first reported the efficacy of immunotherapy by BCG on lung cancer. According to their results, intrapleural use of BCG was effective only for resected stage I lung cancer. However, these results were contradicted by Mountain and his group in their follow-up study.[2]

As an immunotherapeutic agent for the treatment of lung cancer, we have been using OK-432 during the past several years. OK-432 is a drug developed by Okamoto et al.[3] and produced by treating the low virulent Su-strain of *Streptococcus pyogenes* with Penicillin G potassium followed by heating at 45°C. It was first used for injection into tumor sites because of its cytocidal activity exerted by direct contact with tumor cells, the so-called RNA effect.[4] But thereafter it attracted attention because of its host-mediated antitumor effect due to stimulation of the immune system of the host.

During a pilot study, OK-432 was injected into lung cancer patients in the various phases of cancer treatment, such as preoperative, postoperative, during radiation therapy or during chemotherapy. OK-432 injection enhanced cell-immunity, which was manifested in delayed hypersensitivity skin reactions and lymphoblastogenesis which occurred in both operable or inoperable cases.[5]

In 1975, a randomized control study on lung cancer was started to evaluate the clinical significance of immunotherapy by OK-432 as an adjuvant in the treatment of lung cancer.

Materials and methods

Patients

At the time of admission to our Surgical Department, the patients were randomized into two groups, one which was treated by chemotherapy alone (the control group), and one which was treated by chemotherapy plus OK-432 therapy (the immunotherapy group). From 1975 to 1982, there were 342 cases eligible for evaluation of survival rate, 171 in the immunotherapy group and 171 in the control group. The immunotherapy group consisted of 124 cases who had undergone resection and 47 cases who had not. The control group consisted of 123 resection cases and 48 without resection. Staging of the patients was done by the TNM classification proposed by UICC in 1978.

Chemotherapy

For each case, a fixed protocol of chemotherapy was used with a combination of three or four kinds of drugs, selected in accordance with the histological cell type of the cancer involved (Fig. l). For adenocarcinoma and large cell carcinoma, cyclophosphamide, adriamycin, and 5-fluorouracil (5-FU) were combined. For epidermoid carcinoma, carbazilquinone, adriamycin, and 5-FU were combined. For epidermoid carcinoma, carbazilquinone, adriamycin, and 5-FU were combined. For small cell carcinoma, cyclophosphamide, vincristine, methotrexate, and adriamycin were combined. For the cases who had undergone resection, chemotherapy was started three weeks after surgery, and was performed intermittently once every three months in the first year and once every six months in the second and third years. In the cases without resection, the same program was repeated every six weeks.

Immunotherapy

The streptococcal preparation, OK-432, was used as the immunotherapeutic agent. A KE (Klinische Einheit) unit was used to express the strength of the preparation. One KE corresponds to 0.1 mg dried streptococci. Immunotherapy was initiated shortly after the patients' admission and randomization. Administration of OK-432 was by intramuscular injection in all cases and started with a dose of 0.2 KE. This dose was increased at two day intervals in the sequence of 0.2 KE, 0.5 KE, 1.0 KE, and 2.0 KE. The maintenance dose was 2.0 KE once a week, and it was continued for more than three years unless death occurred. About 80% of the patients complained of fever on the day when OK-432 was injected. The grade and incidence of fever gradually decreased as the injections were repeated.

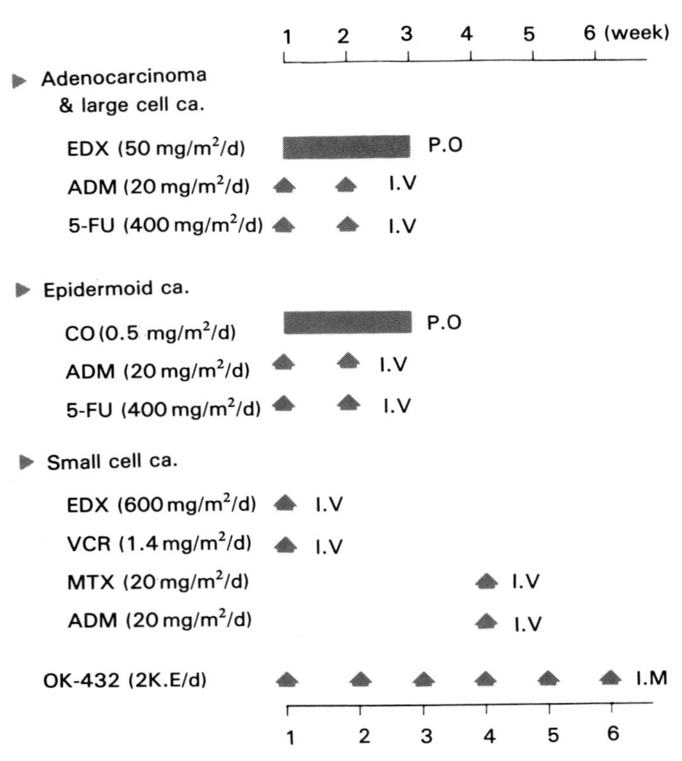

FIGURE 1 *Schedules of immunotherapy for each cell type of lung cancer.* EDX, Cyclophosphamide. ADM, Adriamycin. 5-FU, 5-fluorouracil. CQ, Carbazilquinone. VCR, Vincristine. MTX, Methotrexate. P.O., per oral administration. I.V., intravenous injection. I.M., intramuscular injection.

Monitoring immunological status

To monitor the immunological status of the patients under immunotherapy, the Su-polysaccharide skin test was used in addition to routine parameters such as lymphoblastogenesis, PPD-, PHA-, or DNCB-skin test. Su-polysaccharide (Su-PS), which contains 8% protein, is an extract taken from the cell wall fraction of an incubated Su-strain of *Streptococcus pyogenes*. The reaction to it is thought to be a kind of delayed hypersensitivity skin test.[6] An injection of 0.1 ml (20 μg) was given intradermally, and after 24 hours the longest and shortest diameters of the erythema were averaged. The skin test was judged to be positive if the mean diameter was over 10 mm.

Statistical analysis

The chi-square (x^2) test was used to evaluate the patients' background factors. At the end of March, 1983, the survival rate was calculated by the Kaplan and Meier method,[7] and its statistical significance was evaluated by the Cox and Mantel method.[8] For statistical judgement, the significance level was adopted unless otherwise indicated.

Results

Survival rate by total cases in each group

Table 1 shows a comparison of the clinical background factors of the immunotherapy and control groups. By the chi-square test, the background

TABLE 1 *Comparison of clinical background factors of whole cases in immunotherapy group OK-432 (+) and in the control group OK-432 (−)*

Factor	OK-432(+)	OK-432(−)	X_0^2-value
1. Age			
−29	1	3	
30−39	3	2	
40−49	14	17	2.977
50−59	53	43	(df = 5)
60−69	74	75	N.S.
70−	26	31	
2. Sex			0.404
Male	128	133	(df = 1)
Female	43	38	N.S.
3. Cell type			
Adenoca.	72	62	
Epidermoid ca.	72	65	6.983
Large cell ca.	6	16	(df = 5)
Small cell ca.	11	17	N.S.
Others	10	11	
4. Stage			
I	46	48	0.917
II	12	9	(df = 3)
III	79	75	N.S.
IV	34	39	
5. Treatment			
Complete resect.	93	92	0.016
Incomplete resect.	31	31	(df = 2)
Non-resection	47	48	N.S.
	171	171	

factors of the two groups were found not to be significantly different in terms of age, sex, cell type, stage, and modality of treatment. When the survival curves in both groups were compared (Fig. 2), all 171 cases of the immunotherapy group showed a more favorable survival rate than the 171 cases in the control group. This difference was statistically significant ($p<0.01$).

Survival rate of both groups in each stage

Comparisons were done between the two groups according to the cancer stage. Table 2 shows the comparison of the clinical background factors of the stage I and II cases in both groups. Because the number of the stage II cases in the immunotherapy and control groups were 12 and 9 respectively, stage I and II cases were combined. The comparison of the survival curves between the two treatment groups is shown in Figure 3. The 58 cases of the stage I+II in the immunotherapy group showed better results than did the 57 cases in the control group. However, this difference was not statistically significant. For stage III, 79 cases in the immunotherapy group showed significantly better results than did the 75 cases in the control group ($p<0.05$) (Fig. 4). For the stage IV cases, the 34 cases in the immunotherapy group also showed better prognoses than did the 39 cases in the control group (Fig. 5). This difference was statistically 'virtually' significant because the p-value was 0.053.

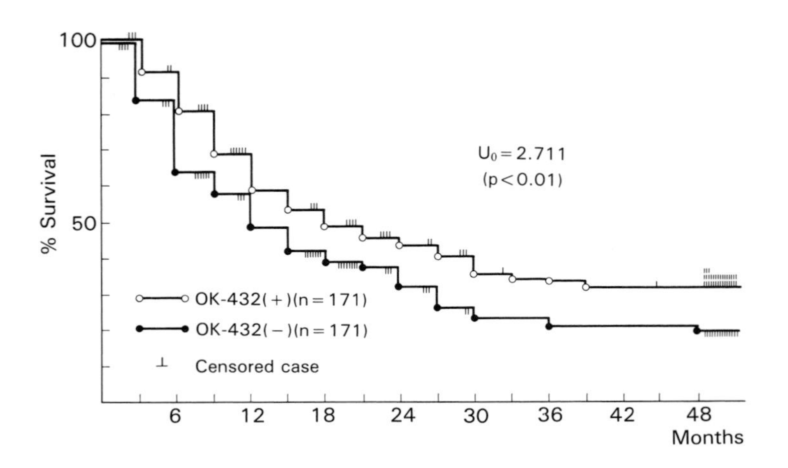

FIGURE 2 *Comparison of survival rates of whole cases in both groups.*

TABLE 2 *Comparison of clinical background factors of stage I and II cases in both groups*

Factor	OK-432(+)	OK-432(−)	X_0^2-value
1. Age			
−29	0	2	
30−39	0	0	7.089
40−49	5	4	(df = 4)
50−59	14	14	N.S.
60−69	33	23	
70−	6	14	
2. Sex			3.078
Male	47	38	(df = 1)
Female	11	19	N.S.
3. Cell type			
Adenoca.	26	27	
Epidermoid ca.	27	18	7.344
Large cell ca.	3	2	(df = 5)
Small cell ca.	1	5	N.S.
Others	1	5	
4. Stage			0.462
I	46	48	(df = 1)
II	12	9	N.S.
5. Treatment			
Complete resect.	53	52	0.001
Incomplete resect.	2	2	(df = 2)
Non-resection	3	3	N.S.
	58	57	

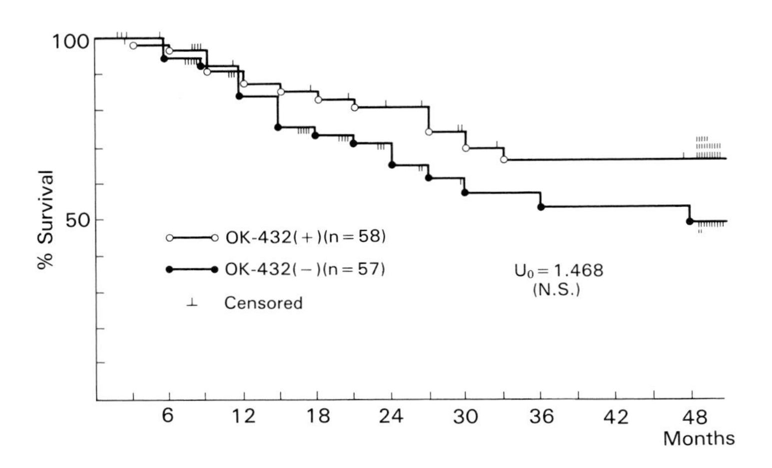

FIGURE 3 *Comparison of survival rates of stage I and II cases in both groups.*

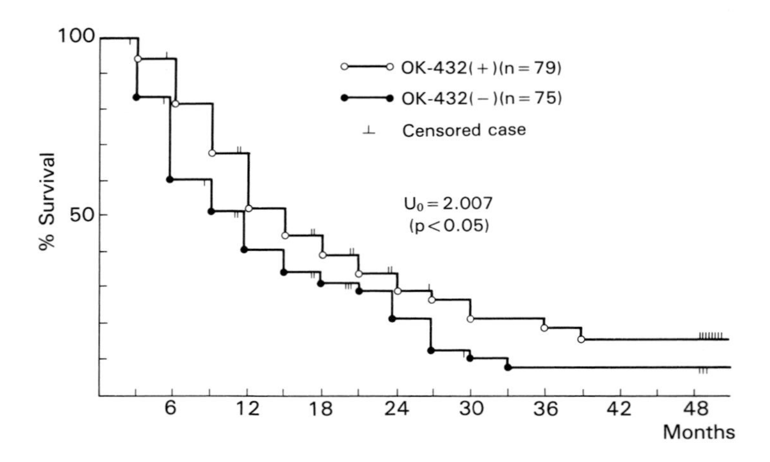

FIGURE 4 *Comparison of survival rates of stage III cases in both groups.*

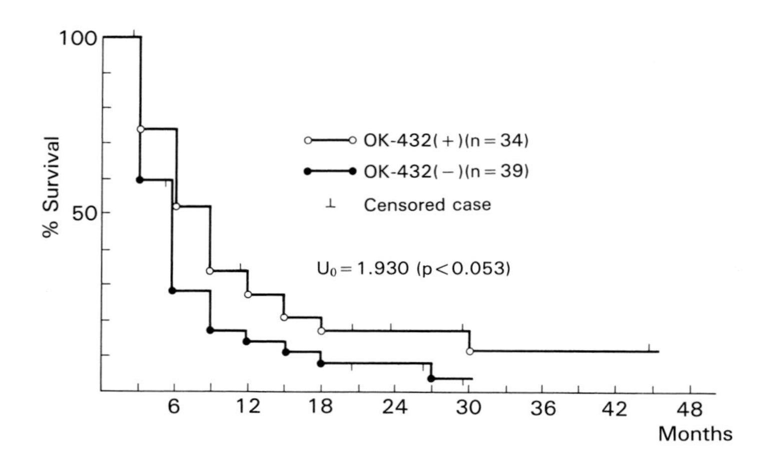

FIGURE 5 *Comparison of survival rates of stage IV cases in both groups.*

Survival rate of resection cases

Table 3 is a comparison of the clinical background factors of the cases in both resection groups. There were no significant differences between the two groups in terms of age, sex, cell type, stage, and operative radicality. The comparison of the survival curves is shown by the solid line in Figure 6. The 124 cases in the immunotherapy group who had undergone resection showed significantly more favorable results than did the 123 cases in the control group ($p<0.05$).

TABLE 3 *Comparison of clinical background factors of resected cases in both groups*

Factor	OK-432(+)	OK-432(−)	X_0^2-value
1. Age			
−29	0	3	
30−39	3	1	
40−49	13	12	6.876
50−59	39	33	(df = 5)
60−69	55	51	N.S.
70−	14	23	
2. Sex			0.109
Male	94	91	(df = 1)
Female	30	32	N.S.
3. Cell type			
Adenoca.	54	47	
Epidermoid ca.	53	48	4.185
Large cell ca.	4	9	(df = 5)
Small cell ca.	4	8	N.S.
Others	9	11	
4. Stage			
I	46	47	0.324
II	9	7	(df = 3)
III	60	61	N.S.
IV	9	8	
5. Treatment			0.001
Complete resect.	93	92	(df = 1)
Incomplete resect.	31	31	N.S.
	124	123	

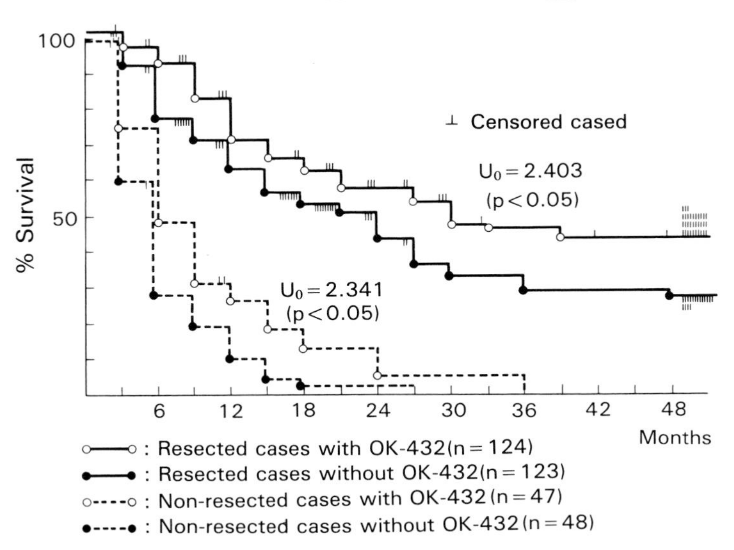

FIGURE 6 *Comparisons of survival rates of resected cases (shown by solid lines) and unresected cases (shown by dotted lines) in both groups.*

Survival rate of resection cases in each stage

Figure 7 shows the survival curves of the stage I and II cases who underwent resection. Although the 55 cases in the immunotherapy group showed better prognoses than did the 54 cases in the control group, there was no statistically significant difference. Figure 8 shows the comparison of the stage III and IV cases who underwent resection. There were 69 cases in both groups. The immunotherapy group exerted significantly more favorable results than did the control group ($p<0.05$).

Survival rate of both groups by operative radicality

The cases who had undergone complete resection of the tumor including

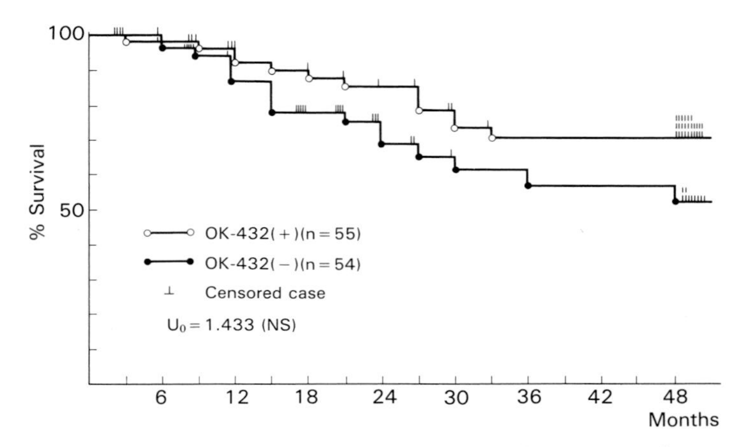

FIGURE 7 *Comparison of survival rates of stage I and II cases undergone resection.*

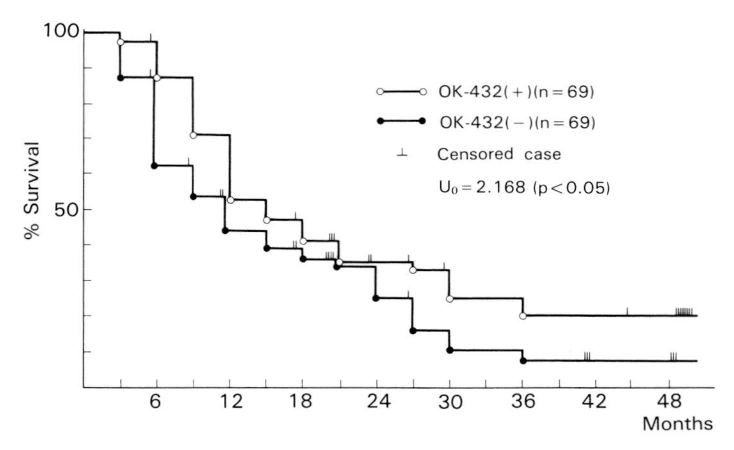

FIGURE 8 *Comparison of survival rates of stage III and IV cases undergone resection.*

metastatic lymph nodes were classified as complete resection. The patients in which the tumor itself, the metastatic lymph nodes, or both could not be taken out completely or the cases of stage IV who had undergone resection of the primary tumor, were classified as incomplete resection. The cases with complete resection contained 53 cases of stage I + II and 40 cases of stage III in the immunotherapy group, and 52 and 40 cases respectively in the control group. Except for two cases of stage I + II in both groups, all the cases in the incomplete resection category were in stage III and IV. As shown in Figure 9, the 93 cases in the immunotherapy group who had undergone complete resection showed significantly better results than did the 92 cases in the control group ($p < 0.05$). Of the cases who had undergone incomplete resection, the 31 cases in the immunotherapy group showed more favorable results than did the 31 cases in the control group. This difference was not statistically significant because the p value was between 0.05 and 0.1.

Survival rate of unresected cases

Table 4 shows a comparison of the clinical background factors of both groups without surgical resection. With the exception of three cases of stage I and II in each treatment group, all the cases were in stage III and IV. A comparison of the survival rates between the two groups is shown in Figure 6. The 47 cases without resection in the immunotherapy group showed significantly better results than did the 48 cases in the control group ($p < 0.05$). These results remained significant when only stage III and IV cases were analyzed (Fig. 10).

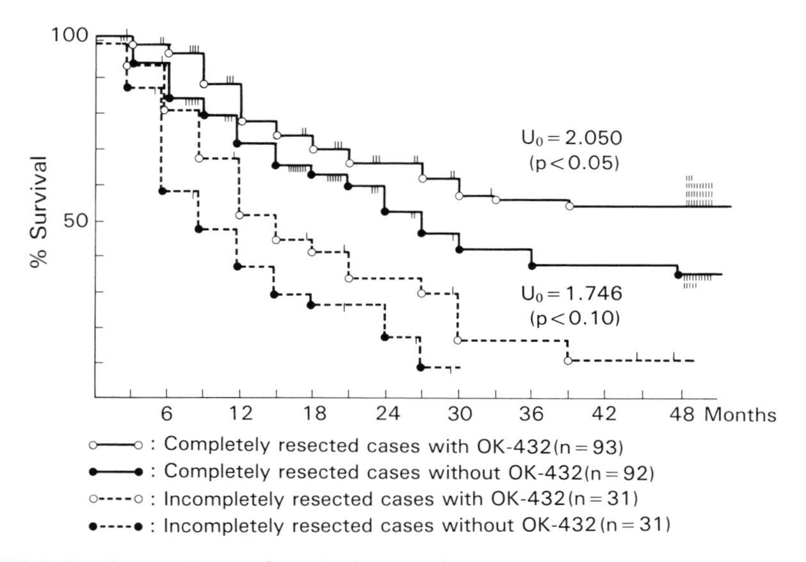

FIGURE 9 *Comparisons of survival rates of completely resected cases (shown by solid lines) and incompletely resected cases (shown by dotted lines) in both groups.*

TABLE 4 *Comparison of clinical background factors of unresected cases in both groups*

Factor	OK-432(+)	OK-432(−)	X_0^2-value
1. Age			
−29	1	0	
30−39	0	1	6.705
40−49	1	5	(df = 5)
50−59	14	10	N.S.
60−69	19	24	
70−	12	8	
2. Sex			3.411
Male	34	42	(df = 1)
Female	13	6	N.S.
3. Cell type			
Adenoca.	18	15	
Epidermoid ca.	19	17	4.402
Large cell ca.	2	7	(df = 4)
Small cell ca.	7	9	N.S.
Others	1	0	
4. Stage			
I	0	1	2.590
II	3	2	(df = 3)
III	19	14	N.S.
IV	25	31	
	47	48	

Summary of the present comparative study of OK-432 immunotherapy

The above-mentioned results of our present comparative study on the efficacy of OK-432 immunotherapy are summarized in Table 5.

Survival rate by cell type

A comparison of the survival rates between the two groups according to cell types was made for the cases with epidermoid carcinoma and adenocarcinoma only, because the number of cases of the other cell types was small. In cases of epidermoid carcinoma, including resected and non-resected cases, the 72 cases in the immunotherapy group showed significantly more favorable prognoses than did the 65 cases in the control group ($p<0.05$, Fig. 11). Conversely, for adenocarcinoma, there was no significant difference between the 72 cases in the immunotherapy group and the 62 cases in the control group (Fig. 12). Statistically significant differences between the two treatment groups were found for the following items: the whole cases, resected cases, and completely resected cases of epidermoid carcinoma; and stage III + IV cases of adenocarcinoma. There were no statistically significant

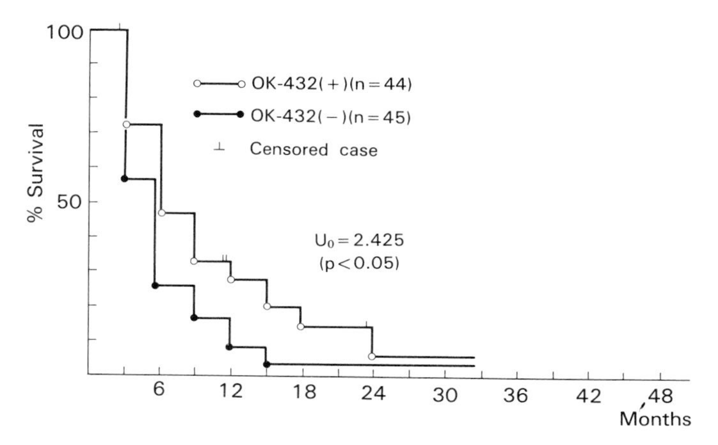

FIGURE 10 *Comparison of survival rates of unresected stage III and IV cases in both groups.*

TABLE 5 *Summary of results of randomized comparative study on efficacy of OK-432 immunotherapy*

	No. of cases		U_0	P	Effect of
	OK-432 (+)	OK-432 (−)			OK-432 therapy
Whole cases	171	171	2.711	0.006	+
stage I + II	58	57	1.468	0.141	−
stage III	79	75	2.007	0.044	+
stage IV	34	39	1.930	0.053	+*
Resected cases	124	123	2.403	0.015	+
stage I + II	55	54	1.433	0.153	−
stage III + IV	69	69	2.168	0.030	+
complete resection	93	92	2.050	0.040	+
incomplete resection	31	31	1.746	0.080	±
Non-resection	47	48	2.341	0.019	+

*Almost significant difference.

differences between the two treatment groups for other items, although the immunotherapy group showed better results.

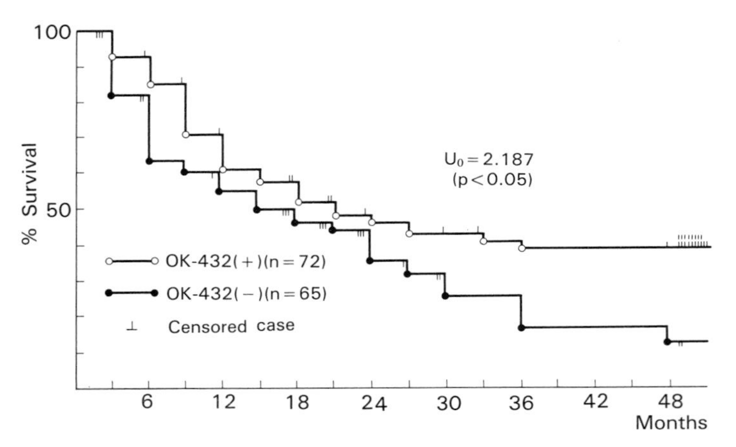

FIGURE 11 *Comparison of survival rates of cases with epidermoid carcinoma in both groups.*

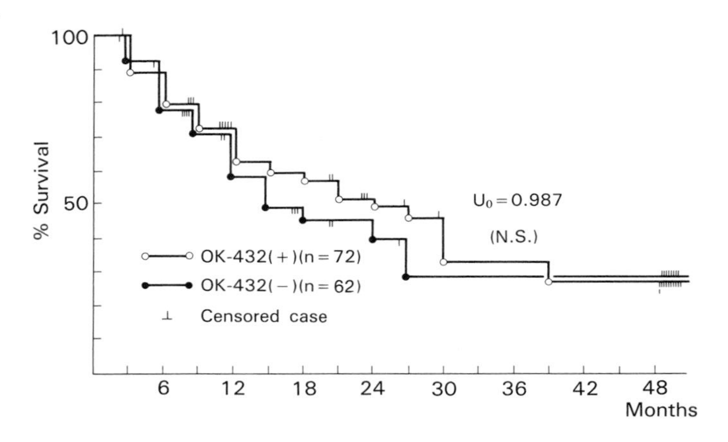

FIGURE 12 *Comparison of survival rates of cases with adenocarcinoma in both groups.*

Su-polysaccharide (Su-PS) skin test and survival rate

When given the Su-PS skin test, healthy persons, non-cancer patients, and cancer patients without lung cancer (most had thyroid cancer and non-advanced cancer of the gastrointestinal tract) generally showed a positive reaction possibly because of a cross-reaction to a previous streptococcal infection. However, most of the lung cancer patients, especially those in the advanced stages, showed a negative reaction. Three to four weeks after initiation of the OK-432 treatment, this reaction was enhanced in most cases. However, in some cases this reaction was not enhanced despite long term administration of OK-432. Figure 13 shows the mean diameter of the

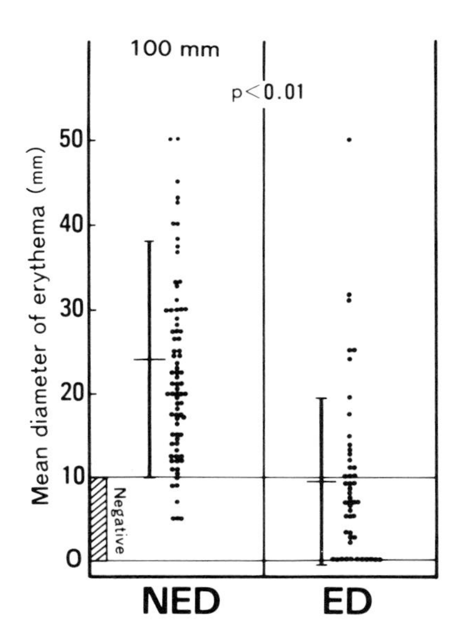

FIGURE 13 *Comparison of reactivity to Su-PS skin test between patients with no evidence of disease (NED) and those with persistent disease. ED, cases without resection, with incomplete resection, and with recurrence of cancer.*

erythemas in the OK-432 treatment groups, comparing the reactions of the patients with no evidence of disease to those of patients with evidence of disease—cases without surgical resection, incompletely resected cases, or recurrence of cancer. Mean ± S.D. of the diameters in the group with no evidence of disease examined in 35 cases was 24.02 ± 13.97 mm, and that of the group with evidence of disease in 29 cases was 9.37 ± 10.06 mm. This difference was statistically significant ($p<0.01$). Figure 14 is a comparison of the survival rates between the patients whose Su-PS skin tests were positive and those whose skin tests were negative for more than three months during the OK-432 therapy. The survival rates of the 85 cases with a positive reaction were higher than the rates of the 43 cases with negative reactions. This difference was statistically significant ($p<0.01$).

Discussion

Since it was first reported by McKneally et al.[1] that immunotherapy using BCG intrapleurally was effective in the stage I cases, immunotherapy for lung cancer has been of special interest. Their method of BCG innoculation was a one-time only instillation through the thoracic tubes of patients who

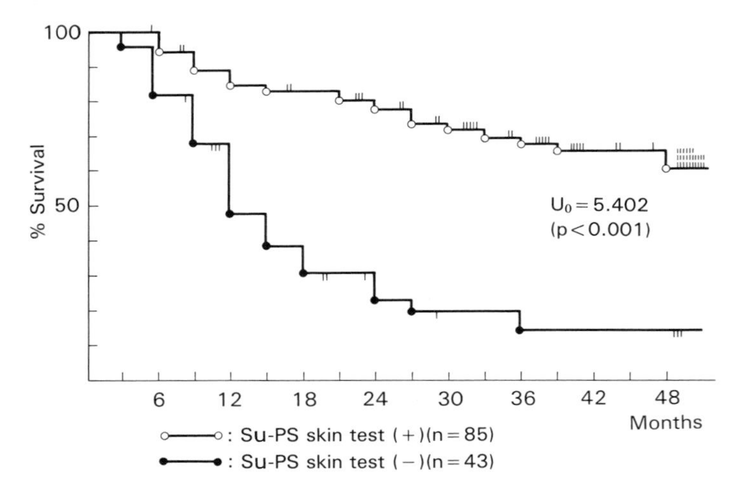

FIGURE 14 *Comparison of survival rates between patients with positive Su-PS skin test and those with negative reaction during OK-432 therapy.*

had undergone surgery. In 1981, the Lung Cancer Study Group[2] tested the efficacy of intrapleural BCG in a double-blind, randomized comparison against intrapleural saline. In a preliminary report, they suggested that there was no beneficial effect of the BCG therapy for stage I, non-small cell lung cancer. In 1981, McKneally et al.[9] reconfirmed the efficacy of intrapleural BCG instillation, but he also mentioned that, at present, intrapleural BCG should not be administered as standard care outside the limits of controlled clinical trials until the question of its efficacy is resolved.

There are great differences between these clinical studies on the efficacy of immunotherapy with BCG and our study on OK-432 with respect to the character of the drug, method of administration, duration of immunotherapy, and combinations of chemotherapy. Kimura et al.[10] demonstrated a significant prolongation in survival time of patients with inoperable lung cancer treated by intramuscular OK-432 in combination with chemotherapy. Uchida and Hoshino[11] reported a randomized comparative study of intradermal OK-432 immunotherapy on advanced, inoperable stage III and IV cases with adenocarcinoma of the stomach and lung. The results were more favorable for the cases treated with immunochemotherapy with OK-432 and 5-FU than those treated with 5-FU alone.

Our present study attempted to evaluate the efficacy of OK-432 as an adjuvant immunotherapy for the treatment of operable as well as inoperable lung cancer. As we have long been using chemotherapeutics for the treatment of lung cancer, this study was done by comparing survival rates between the groups treated with immunochemotherapy and those treated with chemotherapy alone. A maintenance dose of 2 KE was given intramuscularly once a week for three years. The three-year maintenance program is based on the fact that, if no recurrence or metastasis is encountered for three years after initiation of the adjuvant therapy for lung cancer, long term survival of five years or more can be expected.

The overall survival rate in the immunotherapy group was statistically better than that in the control group when whole cases, stage III cases, stage IV cases, resected cases as a whole, resected stage III + IV cases, cases who had undergone complete resection, and those without resection were compared (Table 5). However, there was no significant difference between the two groups in the stage I and II cases, although the immunotherapy group showed a better survival rate than the control group (Fig. 3). The same result was found in the comparison between the two groups of resected stage I and II cases (Fig. 7). These results might be ascribed to the fact that the cases in these relatively early stages show rather excellent prognoses and that there are a lot of censored cases in both groups, so that statistically significant differences between the two groups might be found in future follow-up studies. In fact, our previous report concerning the cases between 1975 and 1979 analyzed in March, 1982, found statistically significant differences between the two groups in stage I and II.[12]

As shown in Figures 4, 5, 6 and 10, the OK-432 immunotherapy was effective even for the advanced stage of the lung cancer. The same results were reported by other authors who used OK-432.[10,11] These results were completely different from the reports of McKneally et al.[1,9] that BCG immunotherapy was effective only for resected stage I lung cancer.

Owing to a limited number of cases in each cell type for precise analysis, it is difficult to make exact conclusions concerning the effect of the OK-432 therapy on each cell type. However, our present study has clarified that the effect of OK-432 therapy was more favorable in cases of epidermoid carcinoma than in cases of adenocarcinoma. This result corresponds with McKneally's report that only the epidermoid carcinomas were affected favorably by BCG immunotherapy.[9] The reason why OK-432 immunotherapy was not so effective in non-squamous cell lung cancer as in squamous cell carcinoma remained obscure. This discrepancy might be related to differences of cell type upon the grade of impairment to the immune system of the host, immunological competence to the tumor cell, mode of extension of the disease, or incidence, size, and growth rate of metastases. Further follow-up studies should be undertaken by increasing the numbers in each cell type and duration of the observation period. In addition a randomized study stratified by cell type will be necessary to clarify this problem.

Mechanisms regarding the effect of OK-432 against cancer cells are becoming clearer because of in vivo and in vitro studies. Okamoto et al.[3,4] who have long been studying the antitumor activities of group A streptococci, reported a direct effect, so-called RNA effect on the tumor cells. Thereafter, many reports of basic studies as well as clinical studies concerning the host-mediated immunopotentiative activity of OK-432 appeared. There is ample evidence regarding the immunostimulative function of OK-432, such as activation of T-cells and macrophages, induction of interferon, activation of natural killer cells, humoral factors, and so on.[13-22] Although the mechanisms of effect of the OK-432 on cancer patients are complicated, the cytotoxic effect of this preparation has two phases: its direct action on tumor cells, and its potentiation of host-mediated immune responses.

Patients successfully treated by OK-432 therapy apparently showed recovery from impaired immune responses. These effects were best monitored by the immunological parameters of cell-immunity. There are many parameters for monitoring the immunological status of patients on immunotherapy; however, the Su-PS skin test is preferred because it correlates well with the immunological status as well as the prognoses of patients under treatment with OK-432.[6] Su-PS is a extract taken from the cell wall fraction of an incubated Su-strain of *Streptococcus pyogenes* and contains 8% of protein. In our recent study, mucoprotein taken from the fraction of the polysaccharide of the Su-strain of streptococci was used for skin tests instead of Su-PS. Close correlation of the results of the Su-PS skin tests and those of mucoprotein skin tests was noted. Most of the healthy subjects and non-cancer patients who were not impaired immunologically showed positive reactions possibly because of cross reactions from streptococcal infections. These two skin tests are thought to be a kind of delayed hypersensitive skin reaction to a recall antigen.[6]

A striking prolongation of survival time was demonstrated in patients who had positive skin tests against the Su antigen during the long term administration of the OK-432 when compared to the survival rate of the patients with negative skin tests. This result indicates that patients immunologically capable of responding to OK-432 therapy might live longer than patients who are unable to respond to the Su antigen even after repeated immunization.

References

1. McKneally, M.F., Maver, C., Kausel, H.W. and Alley, R.D. (1976): Regional immunotherapy with intrapleural BCG for lung cancer. *J. Thorac. Cardiovasc. Surg., 72,* 333.
2. Mountain, C.F. and Gail, M.H. (1981): Surgical adjuvant intrapleural BCG treatment for stage I non-small cell lung cancer. Preliminary report of the National Cancer Institute Lung Cancer Study Group. *J. Thorac. Cardiovasc. Surg., 82,* 649.
3. Okamoto, H., Shoin, S., Koshimura, S. and Shimizu, R. (1976): Studies on the anticancer and streptolysin-S forming abilities of hemolytic streptococci. *Jpn. J. Microbiol., 11,* 323.
4. Okamoto, H., Shoin, S. and Koshimura, S. (1978): Streptolysin S-forming and antitumor activities of group A streptococci. In: *Bacterial toxins and cell membranes*, pp. 259. Editors: J. Jeljaszewicz and T. Wadström. Academic Press, New York.
5. Watanabe, Y., Komori, Y., Yamada, T., Murata, S., et al. (1979): Clinical value of immunotherapy by streptococcal preparation, OK-432, as a postoperative therapy for lung cancer. *Jpn. J. Cancer Chemother., 6,* 811.

6. Watanabe, Y., Yamada, T., Kobayashi, H., Sato, H., et al. (1981): Clinical significance of SU-polysaccharide skin test as a parameter for immunotherapy with streptococcal preparation, OK-432. *Jpn. J. Cancer Chemother., 8,* 1076.
7. Kaplan, E.L. and Meier, P. (1958): Nonparametric estimation from incomplete observations. *J. Am. Stat. Assoc., 53,* 457.
8. Mantel, N. (1966): Evaluation of survival rate and two new rank order statistics in its consideration. *Cancer Chemother. Rep., 50,* 163.
9. McKneally, M.F., Maver, C., Lininger, L., Kausel, H.W., et al. (1981): Four-year follow-up on the Albany experience with intrapleural BCG in lung cancer. *J. Thorac. Cardiovasc. Surg., 81,* 485.
10. Kimura, I., Ohnoshi, T., Yasuhara, S., Sugiyama, M., et al. (1976): Immunochemotherapy in human lung cancer using the streptococcal agent, OK-432. *Cancer, 37,* 2201.
11. Uchida, A. and Hoshino, T. (1980): Clinical studies on cell-mediated immunity in patients with malignant disease. *Cancer, 45,* 476.
12. Watanabe, Y. and Iwa, T. (1984): Clinical value of immunotherapy for lung cancer by streptococcal preparation, OK-432. *Cancer, 53,* 248.
13. Uchida, A. and Micksche, M. (1981): In vitro augmentation of natural killing activity by OK-432. *Int. J. Immunopharmacol., 3,* 365.
14. Uchida, A., Micksche, M. and Hoshino, T. (1982): Effect of OK-432 on the natural killer activity of mononuclear cells in circulating blood and carcinomatous pleural effusion. In: *Immunomodulation by microbial products and related synthetic compounds*, pp. 446. Editors: Y. Yamamura and S. Kotani. Excerpta Medica, Amsterdam.
15. Murayama, T., Sakai, S., Ryoyama, K. and Koshimura, S. (1982): Studies of the properties of the streptococcal preparation, OK-432, as an immunopotentiator. II. Mechanism of macrophage activation by OK-432. *Cancer Immunol. Immunother., 12,* 141.
16. Saito, M., Ebina, T., Koi, M., Yamaguchi, T., et al. (1982): Induction of interferon-gamma in mouse spleen cells by OK-432, a preparation of streptococcus pyogenes. *Cell. Immunol., 68,* 187.
17. Uchida, A. and Hoshino, T. (1980): Reduction of suppressor cells in cancer patients treated with OK-432 immunotherapy. *Int. J. Cancer, 26,* 401.
18. Kondo, M., Kato, H., Yoshikawa, T., Katano, M., et al. (1982): Clinical evaluation of anticancer activity of streptococcal preparation OK-432 (Picibanil). In: *Bacteria and cancer,* pp. 415. Editors: J. Jeljaszewcz, G. Pulverer and W. Roszkowski. Academic Press, London.
19. Koshimura, S., Ryoyama, K., Ogawa, H., Yamamoto, A., et al. (1977): Antitumor activity of protoplast membrane from group A streptococcus. *Jpn. J. Exp. Med., 47,* 341.
20. Natsume-Sakai, S., Ryoyama, K., Koshimura, S. and Migita, S. (1976): Studies on the properties of a streptococcal preparation OK-432 (NSC-B116209) as an immunopotentiator. I. Activation of serum complement components and peritoneal exsudate cells by group A streptococcus. *Jpn. J. Exp. Med., 46,* 123.
21. Ryoyama, K., Natsume-Sakai, S., Hirota, R. and Koshimura, S. (1981): Reduced antitumor and biological activities of the subcellular fractions from group A streptococcus. *Jpn. J. Ext. Med., 51,* 335.
22. Ryoyama, K., Murayama, T. and Koshimura, S. (1979): Effect of OK-432 on immunization with Mitomycin C-treated L1210 cells. *Gann, 70,* 75.

In vivo effects of OK-432 (picibanil) therapy in patients with lung cancer

ALEKSANDAR DUJIĆ[1], VUKAŠIN DANGUBIĆ[2], DESA LILIĆ[1] and NADA KOLASINOVIĆ[1]

[1]Institute for Experimental Medicine and [2]Institute for Lung Diseases, Military Medical Academy, Belgrade, Yugoslavia

Immunomodulation in the treatment of malignant tumors is a provocative and promising challenge, and currently the interest of many clinical trials.[1] Bacterial products have been recognized as potent immunobiological response modifiers which augment immune responses through various mechanisms while producing different clinical effects, and undoubtly merit further study. Among these, a promising agent, picibanil (OK-432) (Chugai Pharmaceutical Co. Ltd., Tokyo, Japan), derived from a low virulent strain of *Streptococcus pyogenes,* has produced interesting effects in trials conducted in patients with a malignant disease.[2,3,4] Our investigations were concerned with the effect of OK-432 on clinical and immunological parameters in patients with lung cancer.

Patients and methods

Our study included patients undergoing radical surgical removal of lung cancer of different histological types (except small cell carcinoma) in the first stage of the disease, i.e. without regional lymph node involvement or distant metastases ($T_1N_0M_0$ and $T_2N_0M_0$). This type and stage of carcinoma was chosen because, according to contemporary medical doctrines, following radical surgical removal of the malignancy, no further radio-therapy or chemotherapy is indicated. This allows evaluation of the effect of immunotherapy (IT) in patients where the administration of OK-432 is the only parameter varied between the experimental and control group, while fulfilling moral and ethical medical criteria. During this clinical trial, patients received no other medication, and, if a recurrence of the disease was observed, patients were excluded from further study and given adequate treatment. After histological verification of the disease stage, patients were randomly divided into two groups, 20 in each. The groups were age and sex matched (age range 39-78 years, only one female in each group). The experimental group patients were treated with OK-432 which was dissolved with 0.5 ml 1% xylocaine and injected intradermally in three sites of the hemithorax of the operated side. Therapy began in the third week after surgery with a dose of 1 KE (Klinische Einheit, equivalent of 0.1 mg of dried streptococci) on the first day, increasing 1 KE each day for 5 days of the first week. In the next three weeks, 10 KE were injected five days each week. Therapy lasted one month with each patient receiving a total of 165 KE. Parameters of immunological reactivity were evaluated in a longitudinal manner: before the commencement of OK-432 therapy (A), immediately after one month of OK-432 treatment (B), 3 to 6 months after treatment (C) and 1 to 1.5 years after treatment (D). Controls were evaluated at the same intervals. Immunological reactivity was appraised by the mitogen induced lymphocyte proliferation assay of peripheral blood mononuclear cells (PMC) with tritiated thymidine uptake (^{3}H thymidine, New England Nuclear), as described in detail earlier,[5] with mitogens in the following four concentrations: phytohemaglutinin; PHA (Gibco) 100-μl, 50-μl, 20-μl and 12-μl/ml culture, and concanavalin A; Con A (Pharmacia) 135-μg, 67-μg, 33-μg and 16-μg/ml culture. Thymidine incorporation is expressed in disintegrations per second (Bequerel). The results were evaluated for statistical difference by the Mann-Whitney and X^2 test.

Results

Immunological reactivity evaluated by the mitogen-induced lymphocyte proliferation assay showed oscilations depending on OK-432 treatment and time elapsed after therapy. Treatment with OK-432 resulted in an increase of mitogen-induced lymphocyte proliferation compared to pretreatment values, reaching statistically significant increases immediately following treatment (B) and three to six months after therapy (C). At this time (C), the increase is also statistically significant when compared to the control group (Figures 1 and 2). When lymphocyte reactivity was assessed 12 to 18 months after therapy (D), proliferation capacity decreased, tending to reach pretreatment values when mitogen Con A was employed. The control group, not receiving adjuvant therapy, also showed a tendency to increase mitogen induced lymphocyte proliferation, although this increase was less pronounced (especially with PHA), and never reached statistical significance (Figs. 1 and 2).

Differences in survival rates became evident only after the patients had been followed for longer time periods. One year following radical surgical removal of the carcinoma, a higher percentage of the treated patients were alive, (89%) as compared to the control group (78%), but this was not statistically significant. After a two-year follow-up, this difference reached statistical significance, since 70% of the treated group was alive compared to 41% of the control group. Survival in the third year cannot yet be evaluated since not all patients fulfill the length criteria, although there seems to be a diminishing beneficial effect of therapy (Table 3).

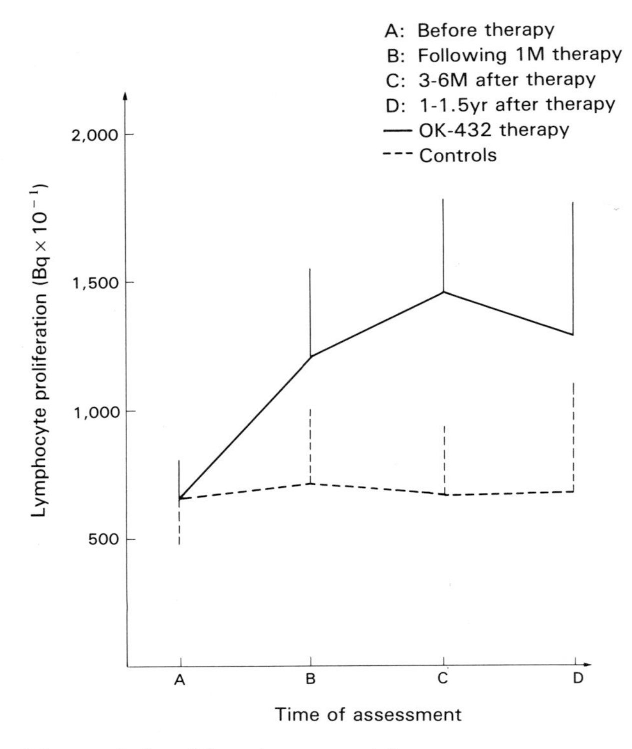

FIGURE 1 *Mitogen induced lymphocyte proliferation (PHA) in patients with OK-432 therapy* ($X \pm SE$).

TABLE 3 *Patient survival with or without immunotherapy*

	Survival %		
Therapy	1 YR	2 YR	3 YR
OK-432	89	70*	60
Controls	78	41	41

*$p < 0.05$.

Discussion

Immunotherapy with bacterial products has already shown beneficial effects in different clinical trials,[1] although a clinical improvement was not always achieved, as we ourselves demonstrated in patients with lung cancer receiving *Corynebacterium parvum*.[6] Katano and Torisu[4] and Torisu et al.[3]

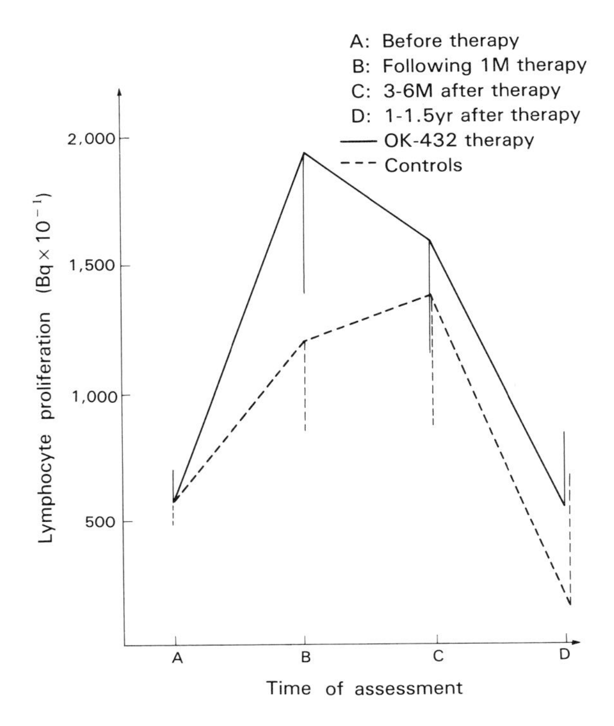

FIGURE 2 *Mitogen induced lymphocyte proliferation (Con A) in patients with OK-432 therapy* (X ± SE).

have demonstrated the effect of OK-432 in malignant ascites, while Watanabe and Iwa[7] presented results of OK-432 treatment of lung carcinoma of different stages, showing significant increases in survival rates. Uchida and Hishino[2] demonstrated a boosting effect of OK-432 therapy on cell-mediated immunity and longer survival in patients with advanced lung and stomach cancer. Uchida and Hoshino[8] found a reduction of suppressor cells in patients with advanced lung and stomach cancer under treatment with OK-432, while experiments performed by Uchida and Micksche[9] demonstrated an augmentation of natural killer cell activity in both normal donors and cancer patients. In evaluating the efficacy of IT many problems must be solved, including correct choice of dosage, length and frequency of treatment, as well as careful selection of experimental designs and control groups for clinical trials. A very difficult task is evaluating the effect of immunotherapy combined with other immunologically relevant treatments such as radio-therapy or chemotherapy, especially when the mechanism of action of the drug in question is still not fully clarified.

To minimize the effects of other factors influencing the effects of IT we have chosen the model presented in this paper, where previously only surgery was employed in the treatment of a malignancy, thus making it possible to have an experimental and control group differing only in one parameter—IT treatment. In such a model we have found that immunotherapy treatment with OK-432 results in an increase of immunological reactivity, as evaluated by the mitogen induced lymphocyte proliferation assay, and in a statistically significant increase in the two-year survival rates of patients under treatment. A definite conclusion on the therapeutic effects of OK-432 cannot yet be given since a longer follow-up period is still needed. Results presented in this paper justify further investigation in this field.

References

1. Spreafico, F. (1980): Current problems with immunopotentiating agents. In: *The immune system: Functions and therapy of dysfunction,* pp.189. Editors: G. Doria and A. Eshkol. Academic Press, New York.
2. Uchida, A. and Hoshino, T. (1980): Clinical studies on cell-mediated immunity in patients with malignant disease. I. Effect of immunotherapy with OK-432 on lymphocyte subpopulation and phytomitogen responsiveness in vitro. *Cancer, 45,* 476.
3. Torisu, M., Katano, M., Kimura, Y., Itoh, H. and Takesue, M. (1983): New approach to management of malignant ascites with a streptococcal preparation, OK-432. I. Improvement of host immunity and prolongation of survival. *Surgery, 93,* 357.
4. Katano, M. and Torisu, M. (1983): New approach to management of malignant ascites with a streptococcal preparation, OK-432. II. Intraperitoneal inflammatory cell-mediated tumor cell destruction. *Surgery, 93,* 365.
5. Lilić, D., Kolašinović, N., Bogdanović, G. and Dujić, A. (1979): The value of some in vitro tests in the evaluation of cellular immune reactivity in a clinically healthy population. *Periodicum Biologorum, 81,* 461.
6. Dujić, A., Dangubić, V., Lilić, D. and Kolašinović, N. (1983): The effect of biological immunopotential agents on mitogen—induced lymphocyte proliferation in patients with bronchogenic carcinoma. *Periodicum Biologorum, 85,* 371.
7. Watanabe, Y. and Iwa, T. (1983): Clinical value of immunotherapy for lung cancer by the streptococcal preparation OK-432. *Cancer, 53,* 248.
8. Uchida, A. and Hoshino, T. (1980): Reduction of suppressor cells in cancer patients treated with OK-432 immunotherapy. *Int. J. Cancer, 26,* 401.
9. Uchida, A. and Micksche, M. (1981): In vitro augmentation of natural killing activity by OK-432. *Int. J. Immunopharmac., 3,* 365.

Review on picibanil special session

Dr. Hirasaka: Dr. Hoshino, Dr. Chirigos and Dr. Uchida, thank you very much for contributing your valuable time, despite the fact that you must be very tired from your participation in the special session on OK-432 this afternoon. Throughout the conference, I have been deeply impressed by the fact that there has been such remarkable progress in elucidating the mechanism of action of OK-432 and by the fact that the presentations delivered today included several studies conducted by investigators from outside Japan. Such interaction was quite unimaginable even a few years ago. The objective of my interview is just to get your impression of the conference itself. Namely, I would much appreciate it if you could give your impression of the presentations or comments on the conference itself from a general standpoint, or make suggestions as to what kind of studies should be conducted in the future in order to establish the position of OK-432 as a potent biological response modifier which can be applied practically in the treatment of cancer patients. Dr. Hoshino, do you have any comments?

Dr. Hoshino: Today's session was very active and many doctors gave open and honest opinions. It seems to me that there were three important topics brought up or clarified at this session. One was the existence of some special lymphokine-like humoral activity which is produced by lymphocytes stimulated by OK-432. This substance is very active in augmenting NK activity or other immunological functions of the host defense mechanisms against cancer. The second topic was that OK-432 can give autologous tumor-cell killing activity to own NK cell population. This kind of activity is very difficult to produce with interferon, but OK-432 does produce own fresh tumor-cell killing, which is the most important issue for the treatment of cancer. The third point, which was less defined, was the question of how long OK-432 treatment or immunotherapy should be continued. In the last discussion, it was noted that treatment should be given as long as the patient is alive. Among the many newly defined immunopotentiating characteristics of OK-432, those 3 topics, I think, were the most important functions presented and clarified in today's session.

Dr. Chirigos: I think Dr. Hoshino covered the presentations at the conference pretty well. There were two aspects, however, that I thought were lacking. One is the work that has been done with macrophage activation. Very little data was presented about macrophage activation. And, it is one of the two most important cells for surveillance not only in cancer, but also in viral and bacterial infections. I think there should be some additional work done with OK-432 and its effect on macrophage reactivity. The other aspect is the question of the administration of OK-432, (how/often and how much). I don't think that it would be advantageous to try to find this out in your clinical study groups because it may be, that you may be selecting the wrong time or the wrong duration of treatment. I think a lot of these questions can be answered with acceptable tumor system models together with the information collected from the clinical applications. And, as Dr. Hoshino mentioned there wasn't any presentation dealing with the treatment of OK-432 on the human tumor where there was any detrimental effect due to the OK-432 treatment. If anything, it was an advantage. I think, the OK-432 meeting itself, was very informative, in that people were very honest about the interaction with the data, and also questions were raised that we will have to deal with in developing the future treatment protocols. The whole congress, the presentations of chemotherapy or bacterial and viral-infections and cancer, of course, dealt with specific chemical entities. The question was raised about the identity of the chemical structure of the OK-432 preparation that has been used clinically. I think that there was just one presentation that mentioned the possible moieties. I feel that some more work should be done on the identification of the components of OK-432. The meeting was very productive and it certainly presented a format as to what directions should be pursued next.

Dr. Uchida: I think there were very good presentations in this session, in both the clinical and research fields. I think that the most important point is whether OK-432 can really augment auto-tumor killing activity or not, both in vivo and in vitro. As I presented, at least tumor-associated lymphocyte cytotoxical activity against auto-anti-tumor cells can be augmented both in vivo and in vitro, and this is very strongly correlated with the reduction of tumor cells in pleural effusion. However, this kind of study is very limited if a cancer patient has no pleural effusion nor ascites, as there is then no means of indication. Therefore, if possible, we should try to obtain tumor cells by operation, maintain them indefinitely at minus 70 degrees centigrade, and use them as the target every month or every week to determine whether OK-432 treatment can really augment this auto-tumor killing activity or not.

Dr. Hirasaka: Thank you all very much. Next I would like to ask all of you a question which is not included in the scenario. I don't think there is wide acceptance of immunotherapy in the United States. In general terms, what do you think about cancer immunotherapy? Is it effective?

Dr. Chirigos: Well, the term immunotherapy to many of us who have been in the field for many years relates to something different than what we are really studying today. This is a new field. Unfortunately, or fortunately, this field has been identified as a field of immunotherapy, however, I would prefer to consider this as an immunopharmacology field because we are now starting to look at the different chemicals that have specific effects on specific cells of the immuno system. And, this is not what was examined in immunotherapy years ago. Today, we are more educated, and we have better assay procedures. I think that it is unfortunate that the tremendous impact we were expecting from the interferon trials has not, as yet, materialized. We shouldn't be discouraged, though. Therapy with immuno-regulators is a new form of treatment and can be a supplement to chemotherapy, surgery or irradiation. I think with enough work in this area of treatment, it will be successful. We just have to keep working at it and trying to determine the important issues about the cellular population that we want to regulate and also the pharmacology that is involved in these agents. So, I think that the feeling that this form of treatment is going to be beneficial is on an upswing. Not only will it be beneficial for cancer, but for other immuno-deficiency diseases as well as for antibacterial and antiviral treatments.

Dr. Hirasaka: Thank you very much. Dr. Hoshino, as chairman of this session, what do you think about the future prospects of such studies and this conference?

Dr. Hoshino: Today's session clarified the fact that OK-432 markedly augments NK-activity, but not ADCC activity. ADCC is, in other words, more specific than NK. One of the future problems to be studied is how to develop more specific tumor-cell killing with the use of OK-432. Certainly, OK-432 activates general immuno-defense mechanisms, but there is very little or no specificity. Thus, I have always mentioned that we must study a more specific manner of treatment, such as combinations of tumor cells with the effective component of OK-432. Dr. Chirigos has already noted some of the other future problems. I agree that OK-432 should be tried not only for malignant diseases but also for non-malignant but very difficult immuno-deficiency diseases, such as acquired immuno-deficiency syndrome.

Index of authors

Subject index